Anatomy, Stretching & Training for Golfers

Anatomy, Stretching & Training for Golfers

A Step-by-Step Guide to Getting
the Most from Your Golf Workout

Phil Striano, DC

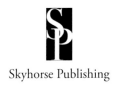

Skyhorse Publishing

CONTENTS

FULL-BODY ANATOMY

FRONT

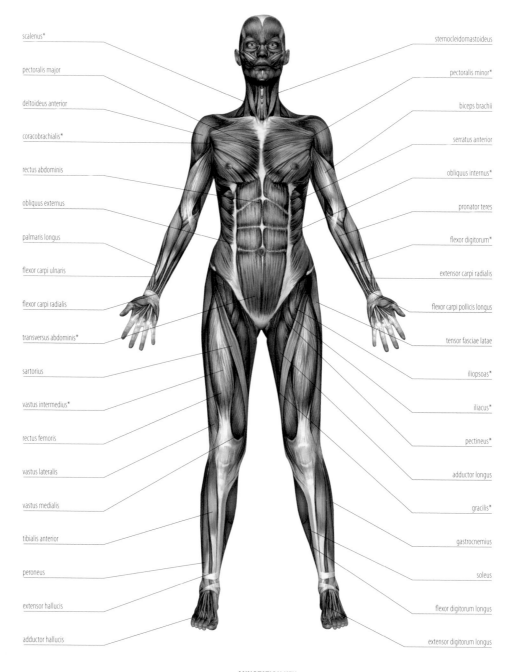

scalenus*

pectoralis major

deltoideus anterior

coracobrachialis*

rectus abdominis

obliquus externus

palmaris longus

flexor carpi ulnaris

flexor carpi radialis

transversus abdominis*

sartorius

vastus intermedius*

rectus femoris

vastus lateralis

vastus medialis

tibialis anterior

peroneus

extensor hallucis

adductor hallucis

sternocleidomastoideus

pectoralis minor*

biceps brachii

serratus anterior

obliquus internus*

pronator teres

flexor digitorum*

extensor carpi radialis

flexor carpi pollicis longus

tensor fasciae latae

iliopsoas*

iliacus*

pectineus*

adductor longus

gracilis*

gastrocnemius

soleus

flexor digitorum longus

extensor digitorum longus

ANNOTATION KEY

* indicates deep muscles

BACK

semispinalis*

trapezius

deltoideus medialis

infraspinatus*

deltoideus posterior

teres minor

subscapularis*

triceps brachii

rhomboideus*

anconeus

multifidus spinae*

gemellus superior*

quadratus femoris*

obturator internus*

obturator externus

vastus lateralis

gemellus inferior*

adductor magnus

plantaris

gastrocnemius

soleus

flexor digitorum longus

splenius*

levator scapulae*

supraspinatus*

teres major

erector spinae*

brachialis

latissimus dorsi

brachioradialis

extensor digitorum

quadratus lumborum*

gluteus minimus*

gluteus medius*

piriformis*

tractus iliotibialis

gluteus maximus

semitendinosus

biceps femoris

semimembranosus

tibialis posterior*

flexor hallucis*

trochlea tali

adductor digiti minimi

ANNOTATION KEY

* indicates deep muscles

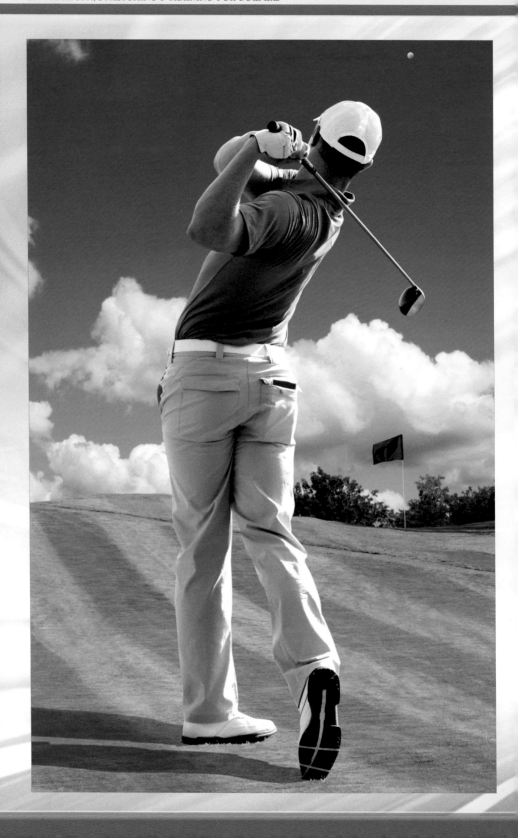

INTRODUCTION: WHY GOLF?

All golfers know the joy they can feel playing the game: enjoying time in the sun, the fresh air, and competing against friends or the course. Hitting a long drive down the middle or knocking your approach shot tight are a few of the joys that make you passionate about the game and inspire you to work toward improving your play.

Most players have taken lessons to improve their swings, with PGA-certified golf professionals, playing partners, magazines and through the Internet. Most of these lessons concentrate on the mechanics of the swing itself. The purpose of this book is to give you a better understanding how your golf swing mechanics relate to your body's biomechanics. In other words, we are going to help you understand the muscles and groups of muscles involved in the golf swing itself. With a better understanding of what your body needs to do during the different phases of the golf swing, you will be better able to train and prepare yourself for the best golf of your life.

As any golfer knows, along with the happiness and confidence that comes along with playing well, frustration and self-doubt come with subpar performances. The goal of this book is to enable you to better understand your body in the swing and play more consistent better golf. Whether you are a beginner to the game or an experienced veteran, you can benefit from stretches that limber up tight muscles, strengthening moves that target your core lower body, and exercises that improve your posture and hone the sense of balance that is so vital to golfing. The exercises in these pages are designed to work a wide range of muscles that come into play when golfing. They can be performed in your living room or office, while striving toward shooting the low round of your life.

GOLF BASICS

GOLF IS A UNIQUE SPORT in that players of varying skill levels, ages and genders can compete against one another on the same course. Golf is also different from most sports in that people of all shapes and sizes cannot only compete in golf but excel at it. Not every person that picks up a set of golf clubs is going to win a championship, but playing confident, reproducible, pain-free and enjoyable golf is a possibility. Golf can be many different things; it can be social, enjoyable or competitive, and it is up to each individual to decide what his or her goals are from this great sport.

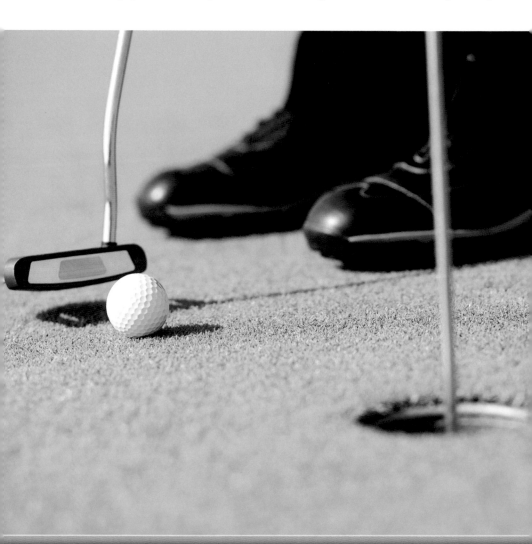

GOLF HEALTH BENEFITS

SURPRISE! Golf does have some physical benefits. Regardless of whether you carry your bag for 18 holes or ride in a cart for 18 holes, you will burn calories playing golf. An average-size man carrying his bag for 18 holes will burn approximately 1400 calories. Walking 18 holes with a caddie carrying your bag will burn approximately 1200 calories, and just playing 18 holes while riding in a cart will burn approximately 800 calories. So as long as you watch what you eat and drink at the halfway house, golf can help you lose weight and stay in shape when played frequently.

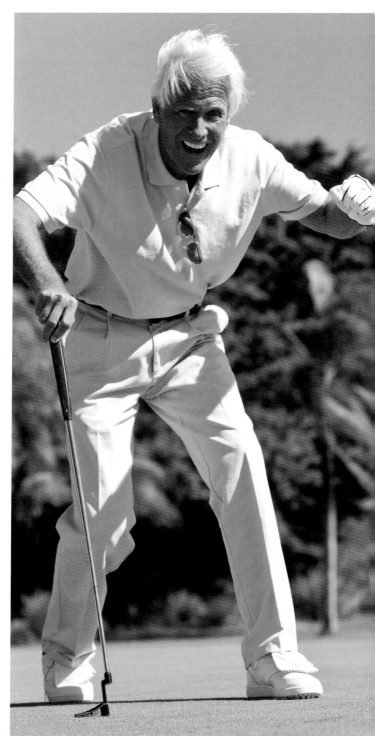

GETTING READY TO PLAY

SAFETY FIRST! Although these safety tips may seem to be common sense for most experienced players, for beginners, it will behoove you to follow these simple rules to avoid injury to yourself or other golfers. Whether warming up on the range or during play on the course, it is of paramount importance to keep in mind your proximity to others. When hitting balls on the range, keep clear space at least four feet in front of you and four feet behind you. This will avoid accidentally striking another person with your club, which can cause severe bodily injury.

Never walk in front of another golfer that has addressed his or her ball. When a player has addressed the ball, he or she will be looking down and will not see you.

Always be aware of your surroundings. Be aware of the group in front of you; do not hit your shot until you are positive that they are not in your range with the club you are hitting. If you do accidentally hit into a group in front of you or to the side of you, make sure you

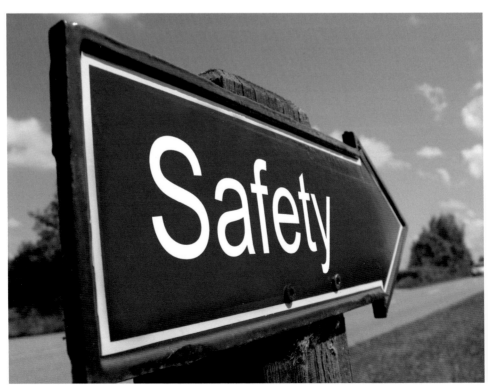

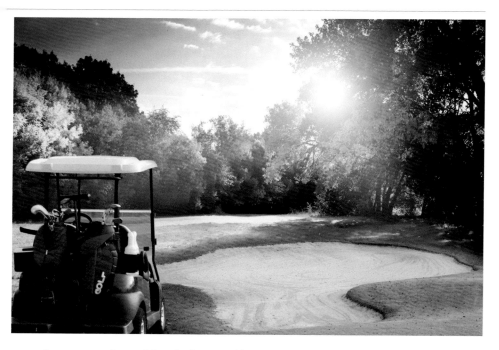

give them an early and loud "fore" call, which will let them know a ball is coming their way and they should protect themselves. Conversely, if you hear a "fore" call from another group, take cover and protect yourself from possible ball impact.

Be aware of the group behind you as well! If golfers are constantly waiting on your group to hit their next shot, they may become impatient and hit up on you. So, for best safety practice, keep aware of your surroundings, both in front of you and behind you.

DANGER
MISDIRECTED GOLF BALLS
NO PEDESTRIANS
MAINTENANCE VEHICLES ONLY
NO EXIT

ゴルフ場内につき誤打球あり、危険
メンテナンス用車輌以外　立ち入り禁止
行き止まり

WEATHER CONDITIONS

GOLF CAN BE PLAYED in varying weather conditions: extreme heat, cold and everything in between. These various conditions can greatly affect your health, safety and quality of play.

Lightning is the most dangerous and unpredictable weather condition that a golfer faces. One should reach shelter when one hears thunder or sees lightning. If shelter is not available, they need to avoid trees, metal and metal structures that may attract lightening. Most golf courses are now equipped with early warning sirens. Theses warning signals need to be obeyed and shelter sought.

Extreme heat and sun are another safety risk. It is very important to drink a lot of fluids before, during and after rounds on days of extreme heat or avoid playing golf during the hottest times of the day. Sunscreen should also be applied, especially for those with fair skin, to avoid the irritation and pain of sunburn. Dehydration can cause dizziness and early fatigue, which can result in higher scores and nausea.

In rainy conditions, be aware of walking on slippery surfaces. Soft golf spikes will give you great traction on the grass but are more prone to slippage on wet surfaces than your regular shoes.

Gusty winds are capable of knocking down trees and limbs, so be cognizant of walking under or around trees that may be susceptible to these winds.

If playing in extreme cold, make sure to layer up your clothing and wear cold weather golf gloves to avoid the possibility of frostbite.

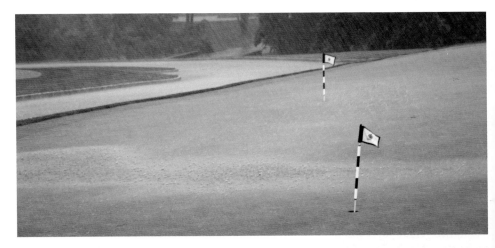

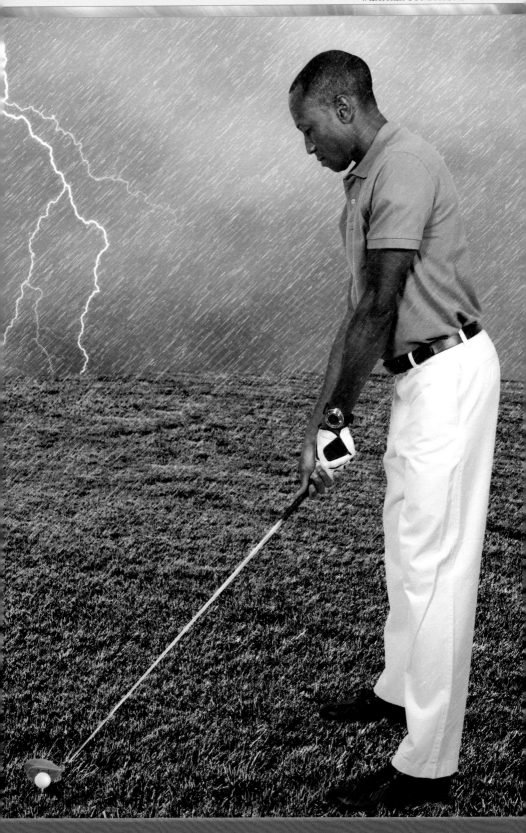

SELECTING THE CORRECT CLUBS

FROM BEGINNERS to tour professionals, choosing the correct equipment is a must for peak performance.

Players just getting into the game can use hand-me-down clubs, or borrow or buy used clubs to begin with, but they should have a wood, some irons and a putter in their set. Going to a local driving range and hitting a few buckets of balls is the first step.

When you feel confident that you are making good contact with the ball,

will consist of three woods, nine irons, a sand wedge and a putter. Fourteen clubs is the most you are allowed to carry in your golf bag for tournament play.

You should be ready to take a few lessons with a certified teaching professional at this point. When you and your professional feel your game has reached a level of skill that allows you to tinker with your set, you may want to take out some irons and add some hybrid clubs and or wedges with varying lofts to fill gaps that may exist in your game.

Your next big step with equipment comes when you are ready to take your game to the next level. If you are shooting consistent scores and are ready to drop your handicap down a few strokes, it is time to go to a custom golf

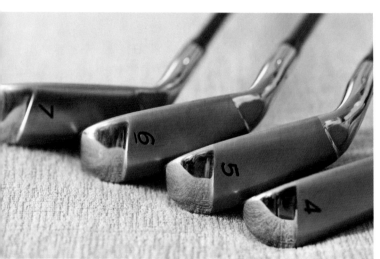

it is time to set out on the course. Start by playing nine holes and work your way up to 18. Do not worry about your score at this stage of the game; concentrate on getting better and enjoying your time on the course.

After having played a few rounds of 18, and hopefully not broken any of your clubs or lost them being thrown up a tree, it is time to get a full set of used clubs. Usually a full set of clubs

fitter. There is a complicated science to custom club fitting that we will not delve into, but we will briefly discuss some of the things they will be addressing with your clubs. Club length, club lie angle, shaft stiffness and kick point for higher or lower ball flight will be assessed. You will be amazed at the fine tuning an expert club fitter can adjust with your swing by making a few equipment changes. The proof will be in your scores.

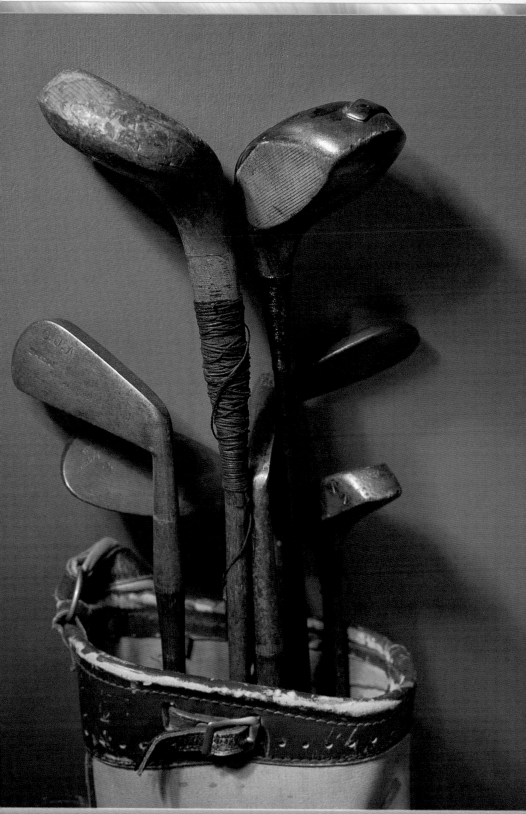

CHOOSING THE RIGHT TEACHER

WITH THE EXPLODING popularity of golf, certified teaching professionals are easy to find. The question is how to pick the right one for you to maximize your learning experience. To answer this question, you need to be introspective. You must find out whether you are a person that learns more through listening or through seeing. All teachers will have different styles. You need to find a teaching professional that matches your style of learning. If you are a better visual learner, you will be better served by a professional that utilizes video capture and playback to teach. Conversely, if you are an auditory learner, you want a professional that explains what they want you to do, a position or set point that they may be looking for or a release point in your downswing. My suggestion for you is to take a few lessons with two or three different professionals to find the one that you are able to "see" or "hear" the best to maximize your time, money and effort spent improving your game.

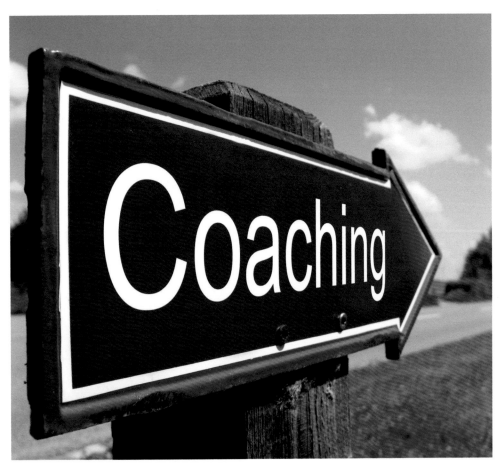

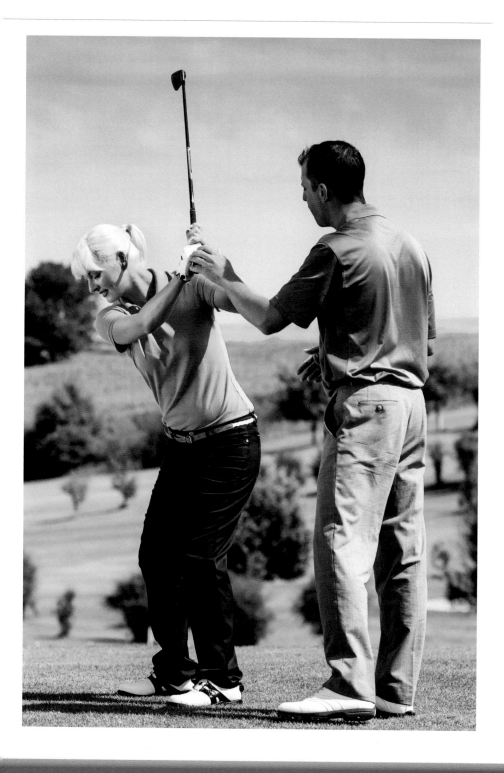

GETTING YOUR BODY READY

WHETHER YOU ARE PLAYING GOLF for the first time or are a seasoned veteran gearing up for a championship season, it is important to put some time into your physical condition before hitting the course. While golf is not the most physically demanding of sports, injuries do occur; however, they can be prevented in many cases.

Preseason golf training is an important factor in preventing injury and should include cardiovascular and strength training, stretching, and proprioceptive (balance) conditioning.

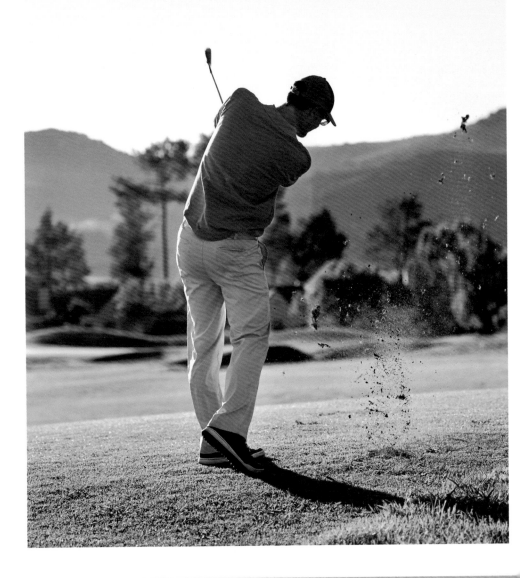

CARDIOVASCULAR:

Since golf is a long-duration sport, lasting at least four hours for casual rounds and even longer for competitive rounds, it is necessary to have the stamina needed to have the same swing on the last shot as on the first. Fatigue can have many negative effects on the golf swing, both physical and mental.

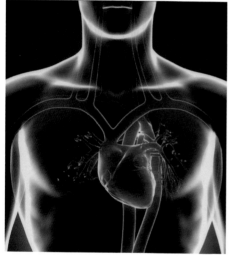

1) Loss of muscular strength and coordination. When you get fatigued, your body will go into an energy conservation mode. The larger muscle groups will not have as much energy supplied to them from your body. In the case of the golf swing, your legs will not have as much strength to hold your balance and fire in the same coordinated motion that it had earlier in your round. Your upper body and arms will become more prevalent in the swing. Fat and thin shots will result from this fatigue.

2) Loss of focus. Your concentration will become dulled, resulting in missing easy putts and poor short game shots that you can routinely make. When a fatigued golfer starts missing on routine shots, he or she will become frustrated. When you are tired, your ability to hit the "reset" button is diminished. At this point, it is much easier to let the wheels fall off the cart then to put them back on!

The average distance a golfer will walk over 18 holes is about 5 miles. Add on a few wayward shots and factor in that courses are being designed longer, you can easily get to 6 miles per round. Depending on your current fitness level, if you have difficulty walking 5 miles at a casual pace, you can most likely expect fatigue while walking 18 holes. Here is how to start a walking/running routine to play fatigue-free golf.

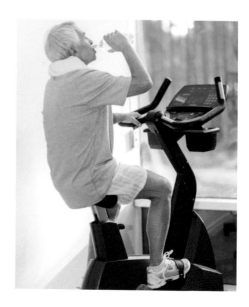

GETTING YOUR BODY READY CONTD.

STRETCHING

We all marvel at the beautiful, long, rhythmic swings we see on the PGA Tour every weekend. One of the main reasons these players are able to achieve these swings is because of their flexibility. Top players work with strength and flexibility coaches to improve their swings. In order to improve your swing, a good stretching routine in the preseason will allow you to play better and more pain-free golf.

When a player has tight muscles and joints, they are not able to get their bodies in proper position to make a good swing at the ball. Sliding, swaying, dipping and lifting up are all swing faults that can result from tight joints and muscles. There are a few basic rules for stretching to gain the greatest benefits and avoid injury.

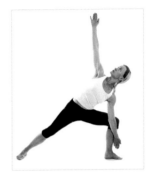

Always warm your muscles up before stretching. Most people have micro tears in their muscle fibers. One is more likely to make these tears worse stretching a cold muscle versus a muscle that has been activated, or warmed up,

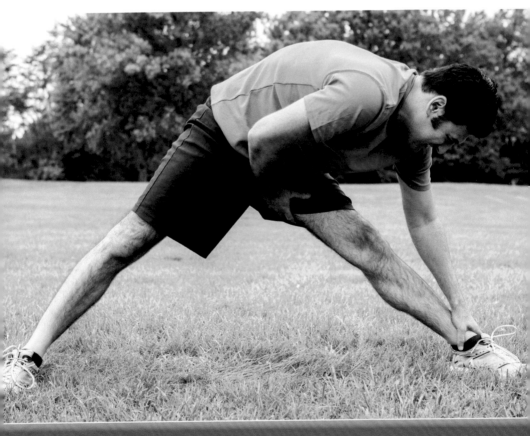

and has blood flowing into it. A hot shower, a short walk, and running in place are a few ways to get your muscles ready to be stretched.

The techniques you employ when stretching are also critical to avoiding injury and gaining maximum benefit. A long, smooth, progressive stretch should be employed. Short, quick, bouncing motions should never be used.

STRENGTH TRAINING

When beginning or altering an existing strength-training program for golf, establishing proper goals is quintessentially important. Muscular strength, endurance and flexibility in the correct balance will improve your game. With few exceptions, the best players in the world, while they work out almost daily with their own personal trainers, do not have large, bulky and tight muscles. Overdeveloped muscles that are seen on bodybuilders and NFL football players can be a hindrance to golf performance. This is because bulky muscles frequently will cause a decrease in an individual's flexibility, range of motion and stamina necessary for optimal golf. This can be avoided by training with lighter weight, full range of motion during the exercise and more repetitions per set.

Since golf is played for 18 holes, doing 3 proper sets with 18 repetitions will help you build strength, increase your muscular endurance and increase your range of motion and ability to use your body's stabilizing muscles. The 18 repetitions will also help you keep focused on what you are training for: playing your best golf!

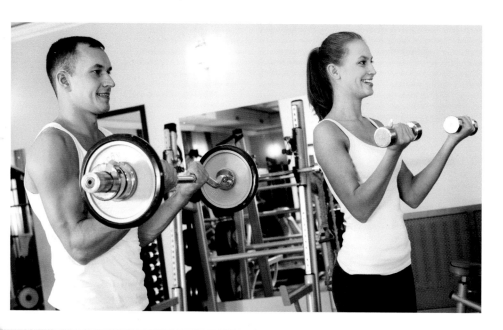

NUTRITION

In order to achieve your goals in sports performance, it is essential to make sure that your body has the fuel it needs to function optimally. In addition to the food you consume, the time relative to your activity—in this case, your round of golf—needs to be coordinated correctly to ensure the fuel your body will gain from the food is available for use.

It will take your body around three to four hours to digest a meal. Therefore, you want to eat around four hours before you play. Since this is not always possible—because of early morning tee times, for example—a smaller meal, which will digest faster, is recommended.

The goal of your meal is to provide your body with the carbohydrates needed to be stored in the liver and muscles as glycogen, which will be released during prolonged physical activity. Good sources of carbohydrates are grains, fruit, pasta and vegetables. Some sports nutrition drinks can also be used to help supplement your body's carbohydrate levels.

The importance of hydrating yourself before, and during, your round of golf cannot be overstated. You should start hydrating yourself two hours before golf and then again a half hour before teeing off. Water or an electrolyte-infused sports drink should be consumed periodically throughout your round. If it is a particularly hot or humid day, extra fluids need to be consumed.

If you become dehydrated, fatigue, dizziness, loss of balance and muscular cramping can result, which will obviously have a negative effect on your performance. Once you have become dehydrated, you will not have enough time to rehydrate your body during your round of golf.

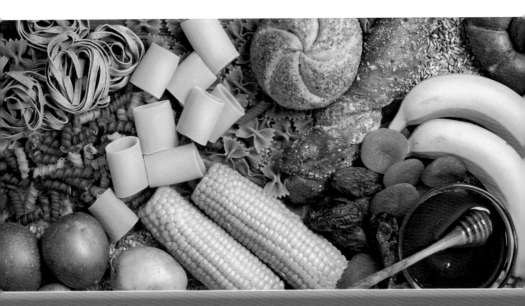

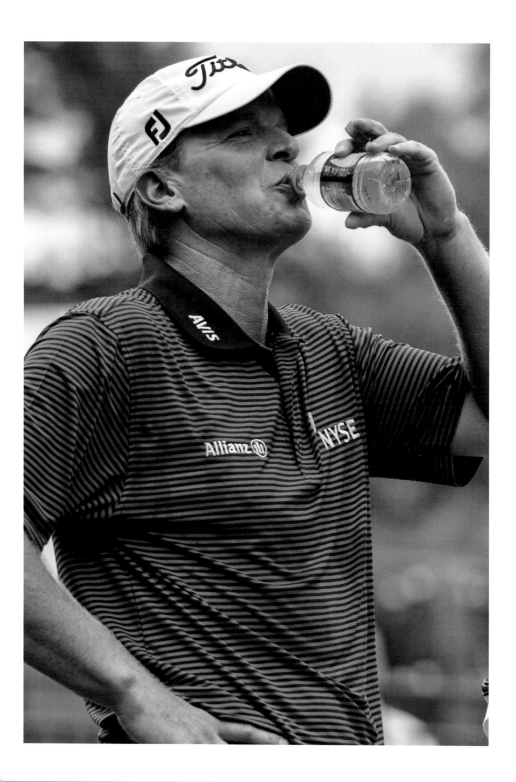

MOST COMMON GOLF INJURIES

TO EXCEL AT GOLF, a player needs to put in a lot of time and practice. The repetitive and explosive nature of the golf swing puts a great amount of stress on the muscles, ligaments and joints in the body. Many injuries can be prevented by properly warming up, and by stretching your muscles and joints before playing.

It is also important to be cognitive of warning signs your body may be signaling to you. Do not allow a minor injury, which may force you to take a little time away from golf, become a major injury, taking months or whole seasons of golfing away from you. Pain, discomfort, and soreness are all signals from your body that something is injured. You need to listen to your body and determine whether trying to play through the pain is making the injury worse. If the pain persists, see a qualified health-care professional to be evaluated, diagnosed and treated properly.

Common factors contributing to injuries resulting from golf:

- Not warming up the muscles adequately
- Swinging too hard
- Poor swing mechanics
- Over-practicing/ taking too many swings
- Repetitive rotational forces to the spine
- Impact forces from the club hitting the ground/hitting the ball "fat"

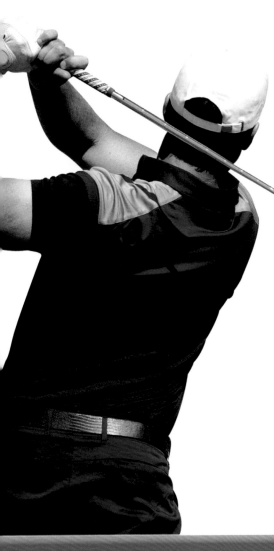

LOWER BACK PAIN

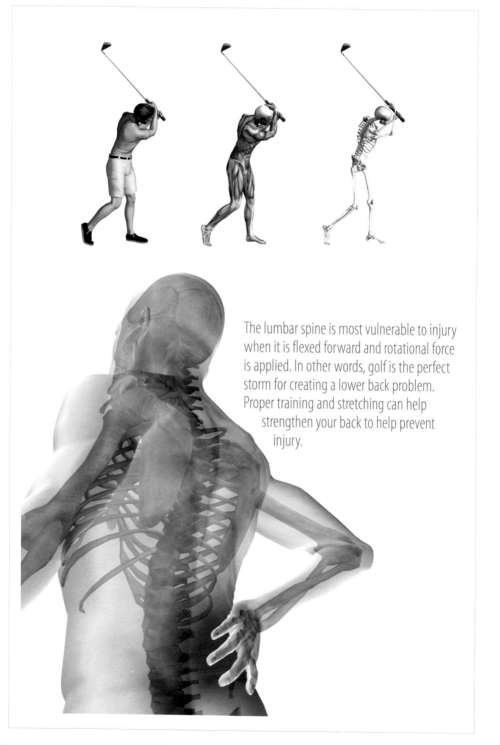

The lumbar spine is most vulnerable to injury when it is flexed forward and rotational force is applied. In other words, golf is the perfect storm for creating a lower back problem. Proper training and stretching can help strengthen your back to help prevent injury.

LOWER BACK PAIN

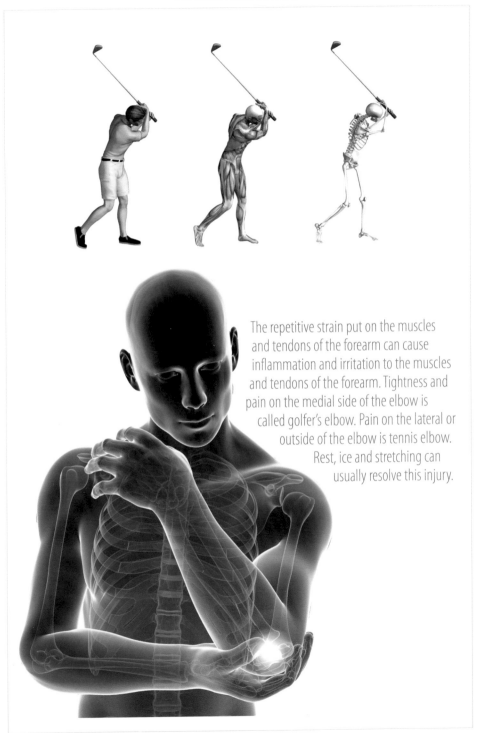

The repetitive strain put on the muscles and tendons of the forearm can cause inflammation and irritation to the muscles and tendons of the forearm. Tightness and pain on the medial side of the elbow is called golfer's elbow. Pain on the lateral or outside of the elbow is tennis elbow. Rest, ice and stretching can usually resolve this injury.

KNEE PAIN

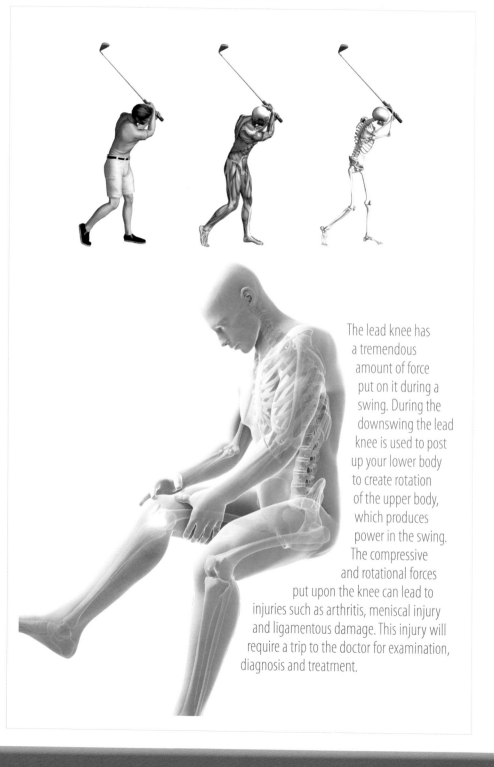

The lead knee has a tremendous amount of force put on it during a swing. During the downswing the lead knee is used to post up your lower body to create rotation of the upper body, which produces power in the swing. The compressive and rotational forces put upon the knee can lead to injuries such as arthritis, meniscal injury and ligamentous damage. This injury will require a trip to the doctor for examination, diagnosis and treatment.

WRIST INJURIES

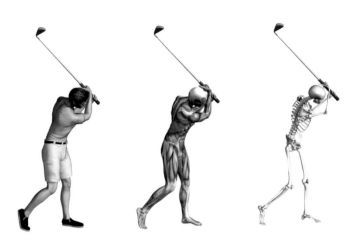

The repetitive strain that is put on the wrist at the top of the swing and also at impact can lead to tendon and ligamentous injury. A golfer that takes deep divots frequently is prone to this injury. Pain, decreased range of motion and swelling would be symptoms related to such injuries. Traumatic injury to the wrist can occur if the club strikes hard and set objects, such as rock and tree roots, on impact.

SHOULDER INJURIES

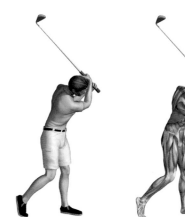

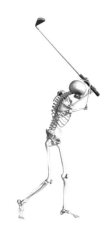

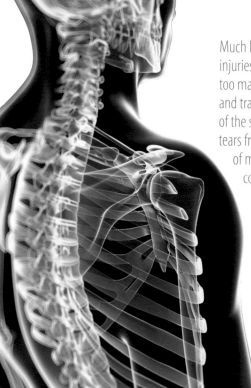

Much like injuries to the wrist, shoulder injuries predominantly occur as a result of too many repetitions, poor swing mechanics and traumatic force. The rotator cuff muscles of the shoulder can develop tendinitis and tears from overuse. Pain and decreased range of motion will be present with these conditions.

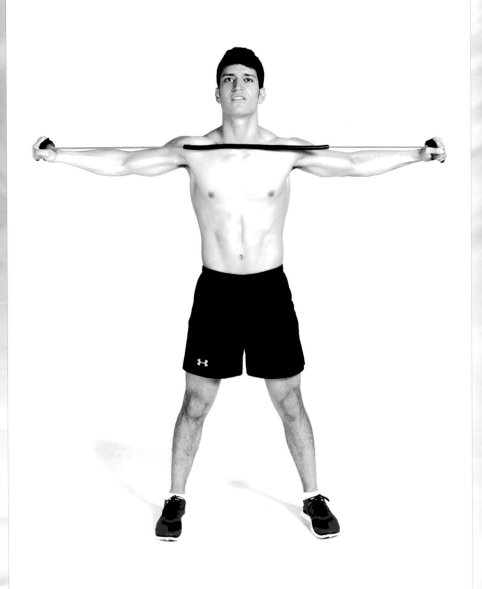

ARMS, SHOULDERS AND CHEST

If you want to increase your swing speed, then shoulder strengthening should be one of the most important parts to your golf work-out routine! Having strong shoulder muscles is essential to a proper golf swing. Elbow injuries are one of the most common golf-related injuries. Making sure that this area is strong is extremely important. The forearms are really the key area to focus on strengthening as they protect you from elbow and wrist injury. You will use your triceps primarily for force-generation during the downswing, and you should exercise your biceps for stability.

TRICEPS STRETCH

STRETCH

THE TRICEPS, the muscle on the back of your upper arm, are especially important to keep loose, as they are vital to a good swing and are used in many exercises in this book.

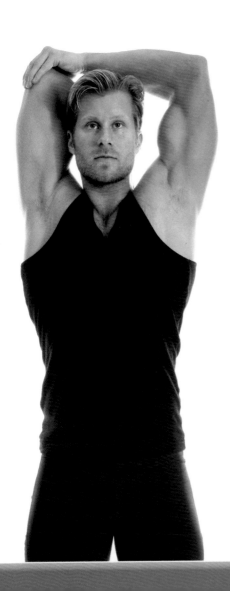

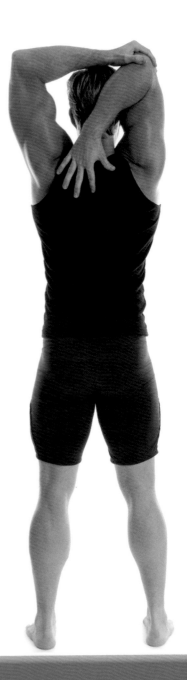

HOW TO DO IT

1 Stand with your legs and feet parallel and shoulder-width apart. Bend your knees very slightly, and tuck your pelvis slightly forward, lift your chest, and press your shoulders downward and back.

2 Reach your right arm up behind your head, and bend it from the elbow, aiming to bring your elbow toward the middle of the back of your head. Your right hand should fall between your shoulder blades.

3 Grab your right elbow with your left hand, and gently pull to intensify the stretch while the elbow stays still.

4 Release your elbow and repeat on the other side.

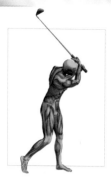

PRIMARY TARGETS
• triceps brachii

BENEFITS
• Upper arms

CAUTIONS
• Tilting your head and/or neck forward, jeopardizing your spinal alignment.
• Holding your breath.

PERFECT YOUR FORM
• Keep your shoulders pressed down and back, away from your ears.
• Maintain a firm, stable midsection, keeping your pelvis slightly tucked in.

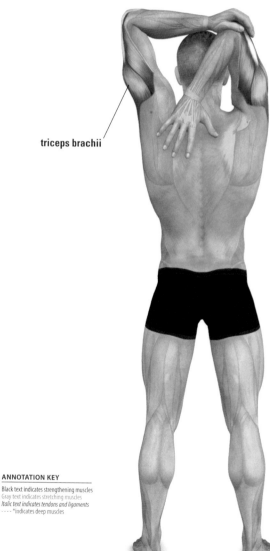

triceps brachii

ANNOTATION KEY
Black text indicates strengthening muscles
Gray text indicates stretching muscles
Italic text indicates tendons and ligaments
- - - - *indicates deep muscles

BICEPS STRETCH

STRETCH

THIS BICEP STRETCH is designed to improve the flexibility of the bicep muscle. Be sure to keep your back upright and your pectorals engaged while performing this stretch—as with most exercises, you work more than just the targeted muscles.

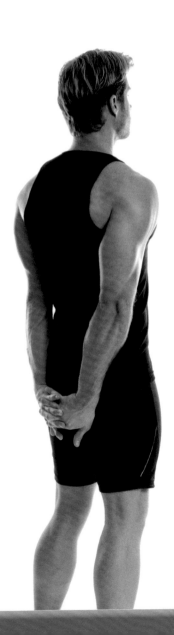
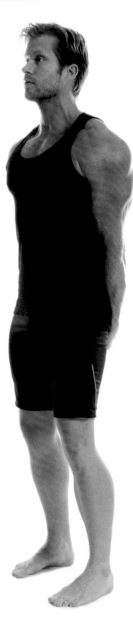

HOW TO DO IT

1 Stand with your legs and feet parallel and shoulder-width apart. Bend your knees very slightly, and tuck your pelvis slightly forward, lift your chest, and press your shoulders downward and back.

2 Clasp your hands together behind your back with your palms together, straighten your arms, and twist your wrists inward, bringing your palms to your gluteal muscles.

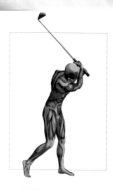

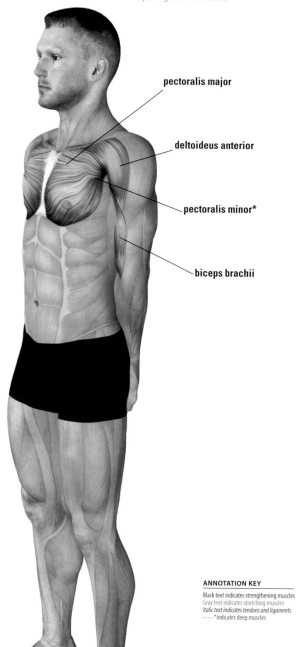

pectoralis major

deltoideus anterior

pectoralis minor*

biceps brachii

PRIMARY TARGETS
• biceps brachii
• deltoideus anterior
• pectoralis major
• pectoralis minor

BENEFITS
• Upper arms
• Shoulders
• Chest

CAUTIONS
• Collapsing your chest forward.

PERFECT YOUR FORM
• Keep your shoulders pressed down and back, away from your ears.

ANNOTATION KEY

Black text indicates strengthening muscles
Gray text indicates stretching muscles
Italic text indicates tendons and ligaments
- - - - *indicates deep muscles

WALL-ASSISTED CHEST STRETCH

STRETCH

THIS STRETCH IS GREAT because it allows you to focus on one side at a time; plus, you can do it anywhere there's a wall or pole. If you sit most of the day or if you commute long distances this is a great chest-opening stretch.

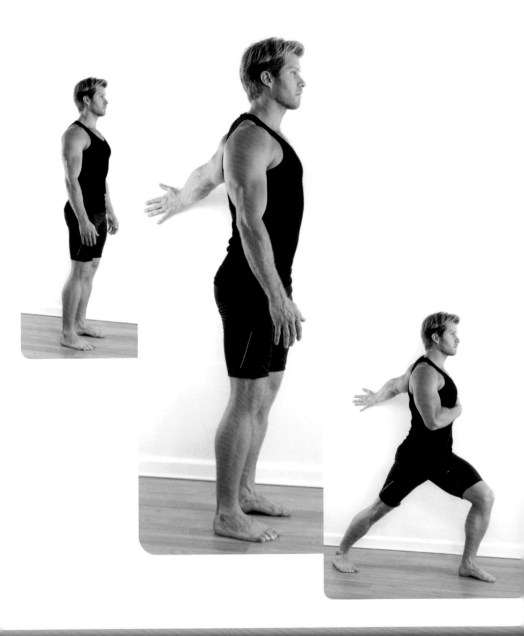

HOW TO DO IT

1 Stand parallel to a wall, with the wall on the left side of your body.

2 Extend your left arm back against the wall, so that your palm is flat against it.

3 Lunge forward with your left foot.

4 Remain facing forward as you stretch. To stay aware of any torso twisting, place your right hand just below your left pectoral muscle, fingers on your rib cage.

5 Return to the starting position, turn so that the wall is on your right, and repeat.

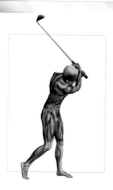

PRIMARY TARGETS
- deltoideus anterior
- pectoralis major
- pectoralis minor

BENEFITS
- Chest
- Shoulders
- Stretches lower back, chest, and glutes

CAUTIONS
- Avoid rotating your chest and/or torso toward the wall when lunging; instead, face forward.

PERFECT YOUR FORM
- Keep your shoulders pressed down and back, away from your ears.
- Position the arm against the wall so your elbow is slightly lower than your shoulder and your wrist is slightly below your elbow.

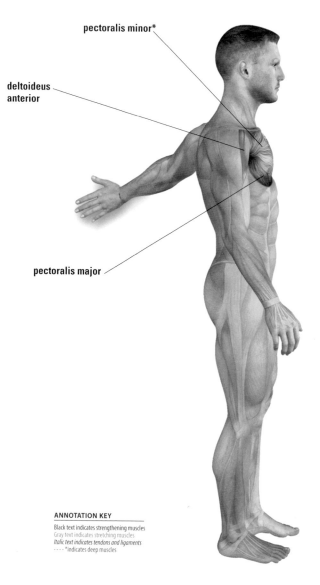

pectoralis minor*

deltoideus anterior

pectoralis major

ANNOTATION KEY

Black text indicates strengthening muscles
Gray text indicates stretching muscles
Italic text indicates tendons and ligaments
- - - - *indicates deep muscles

FRONT DELTOID TOWEL STRETCH

STRETCH

YOU'LL FEEL THIS STRETCH all around your shoulder, but especially in the front part of your deltoid. You don't have to use a towel, of course, a t-shirt or piece of rope will work just as well.

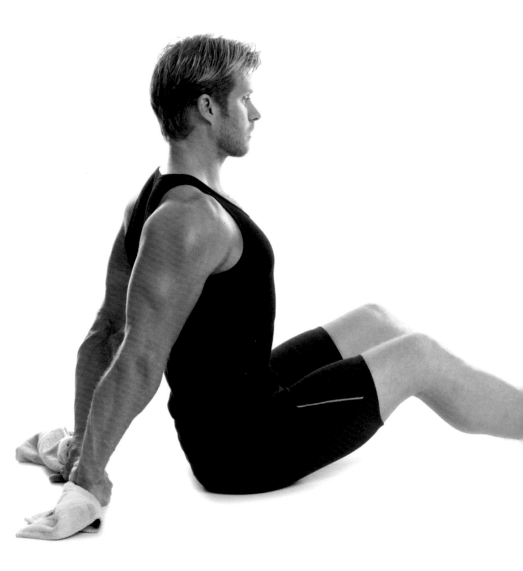

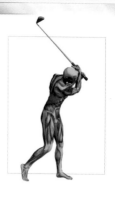

HOW TO DO IT

1 Sit on the floor with your legs extended in parallel position, knees slightly bent and heels on the floor. Grip a small towel behind your back, palms facing behind you.

2 Gently slide your buttocks forward along the floor until you feel a comfortable stretch in your front deltoids. Return to the starting position, and repeat if desired.

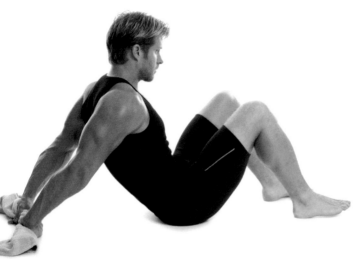

PRIMARY TARGETS
- pectoralis minor
- deltoideus anterior
- pectoralis major

BENEFITS
- Shoulders

CAUTIONS
- Avoid leaning your head forward; instead, keep it in line with your body.

PERFECT YOUR FORM
- Keep your hands together while gripping the towel

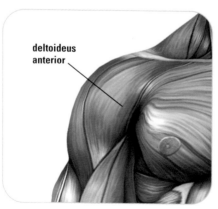

deltoideus anterior

ANNOTATION KEY

Black text indicates strengthening muscles
Gray text indicates stretching muscles
Italic text indicates tendons and ligaments
- - - - *indicates deep muscles

FOREARM STRETCHES

STRETCH

WRIST FLEXION

Perform this stretch after a long phone conversation or a stressful commute to release any tension in your hands and forearms—and, of course, before your round of golf.

WRIST EXTENSION

Imagine that you are holding the eraser end of a pencil under each arm—engage the muscles around your armpits to hold your imaginary pencils, keeping your shoulders perfectly positioned in the process.

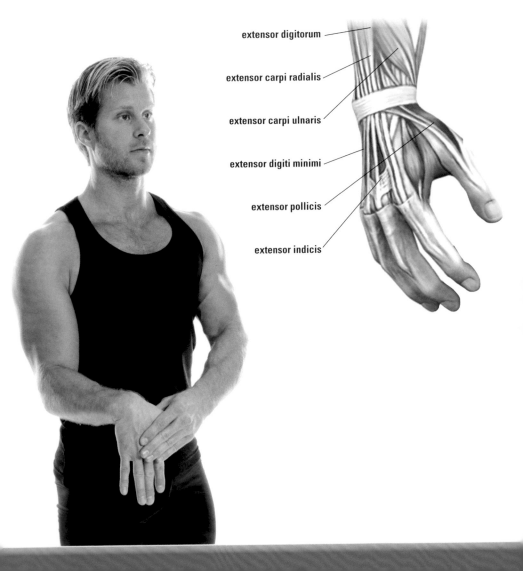

extensor digitorum

extensor carpi radialis

extensor carpi ulnaris

extensor digiti minimi

extensor pollicis

extensor indicis

HOW TO DO IT

1 Stand or sit with your arms at your sides.

2 Bend your right forearm up from the elbow, creating a 90-degree bend. Your palm should be facing the floor.

3 Drop and flex your right wrist downward so that your palm faces inward.

4 Place your left fingers over the back of your right hand and your left thumb on the palm of the hand, directly on the right thumb muscle.

5 Gently press your left fingers into the back of your right hand, bringing your right wrist to a 60- to 90-degree bend, while pressing your left thumb into the palm away from the body, creating a deeper stretch.

6 Release, switch hands, and repeat on the other side.

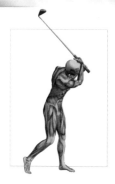

PRIMARY TARGETS
- extensor carpi radialis
- extensor carpi ulnaris
- extensor digiti minimi
- extensor digitorum
- extensor indicis
- extensor pollicis

BENEFITS
- Wrists
- Hands
- Forearms

CAUTIONS
- Avoid lifting or tensing your shoulders.

PERFECT YOUR FORM
- Be sure to press your thumb into the meaty part of your palm, attached to the thumb, intensifying the stretch in your forearm and wrist.

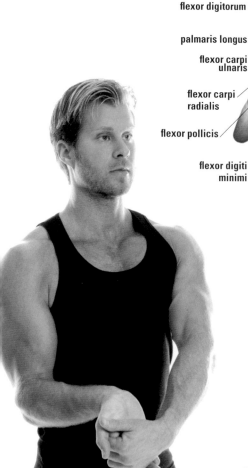

flexor digitorum

palmaris longus

flexor carpi ulnaris

flexor carpi radialis

flexor pollicis

flexor digiti minimi

ANNOTATION KEY

Black text indicates strengthening muscles
Gray text indicates stretching muscles
Italic text indicates tendons and ligaments
- - - - *indicates deep muscles

DIPS

BEGINNER

VERTICAL DIPS ARE A FANTASTIC TRICEPS STRENGTHENER; they also work the entire upper body. An explosive movement, the vertical dip is a well-established exercise that repays its practitioner heavy dividends.

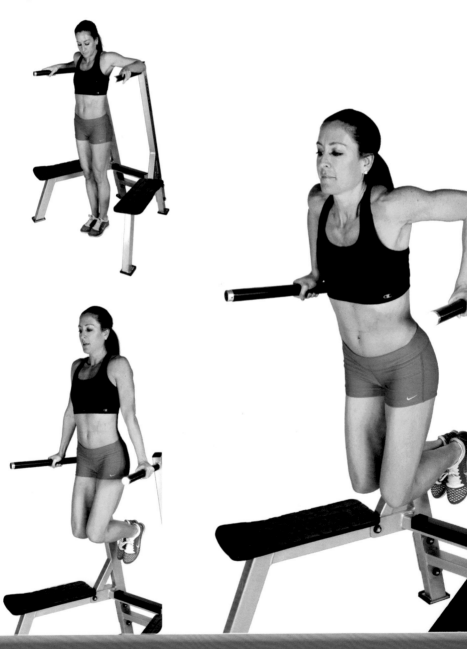

HOW TO DO IT

1 Begin standing in front of a dip station or parallel bars.

2 Place one hand on each bar, and grip as you push and extend your arms to full lockout.

3 Lower yourself until your upper arms are parallel to the ground, then push back up to the starting position. Complete 8–10 repetitions.

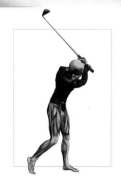

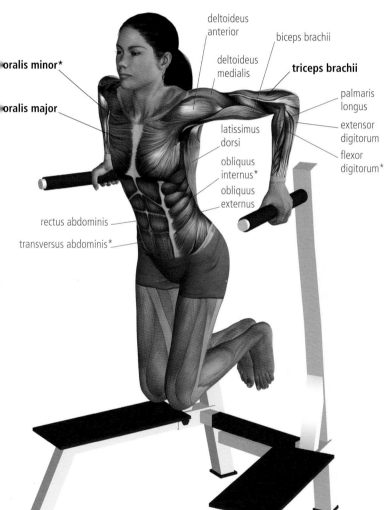

oralis minor*

oralis major

rectus abdominis

transversus abdominis*

deltoideus anterior

biceps brachii

deltoideus medialis

triceps brachii

latissimus dorsi

obliquus internus*

obliquus externus

palmaris longus

extensor digitorum

flexor digitorum*

PRIMARY TARGETS
• pectoralis major
• pectoralis minor
• triceps brachii

BENEFITS
• Increases strength and mass in the upper body

CAUTIONS
• Avoid performing the exercise at excessive speed.

PERFECT YOUR FORM
• Always complete a full range of motion.

ANNOTATION KEY

Black text indicates strengthening muscles
Gray text indicates stretching muscles
Italic text indicates tendons and ligaments
- - - - *indicates deep muscles

BOTTOMS-UP KETTLEBELL CLEAN

BEGINNER

THE BOTTOMS-UP KETTLEBELL CLEAN is a simple way of developing strength in the forearms, biceps and shoulders. Be sure to stand upright, with your feet shoulder-width apart.

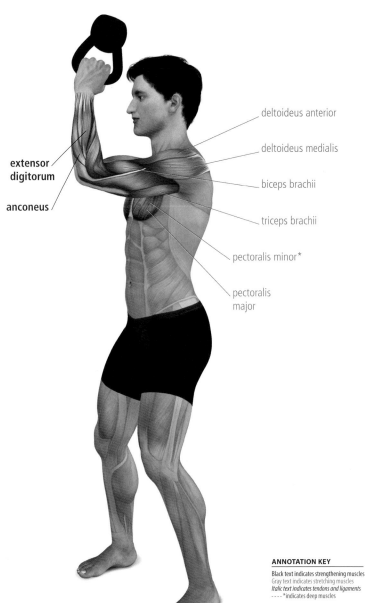

extensor
digitorum

anconeus

deltoideus anterior

deltoideus medialis

biceps brachii

triceps brachii

pectoralis minor*

pectoralis
major

ANNOTATION KEY

Black text indicates strengthening muscles
Gray text indicates stretching muscles
Italic text indicates tendons and ligaments
- - - - *indicates deep muscles

HOW TO DO IT

1 Stand upright, with your feet shoulder-width apart, holding a kettlebell in your left hand. Swing the kettlebell backward, then bring it forward and above your head forcefully, squeezing the handle as you do so.

2 Once your upper arm is parallel to the floor, hold the position, then lower your arm again. Complete 8–10 repetitions before switching to the other arm.

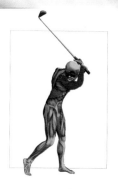

PRIMARY TARGETS
- palmaris longus
- flexor carpi ulnaris
- pronator teres
- flexor digitorum
- anconeus
- extensor digitorum

BENEFITS
- Forearms
- Biceps
- Shoulders

CAUTIONS
- Avoid adopting a loose grip.

PERFECT YOUR FORM
- Keep your back straight throughout the movement.

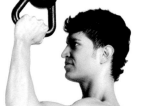

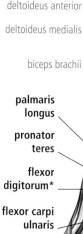

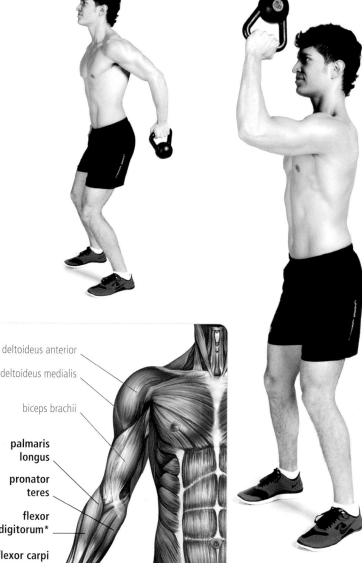

deltoideus anterior

deltoideus medialis

biceps brachii

palmaris longus

pronator teres

flexor digitorum*

flexor carpi ulnaris

BAND PULL-APART

BEGINNER

THE BAND PULL-APART is a simple routine that targets the middle back, trapezius and shoulders. It is a straightforward way of increasing strength and mass in your shoulders.

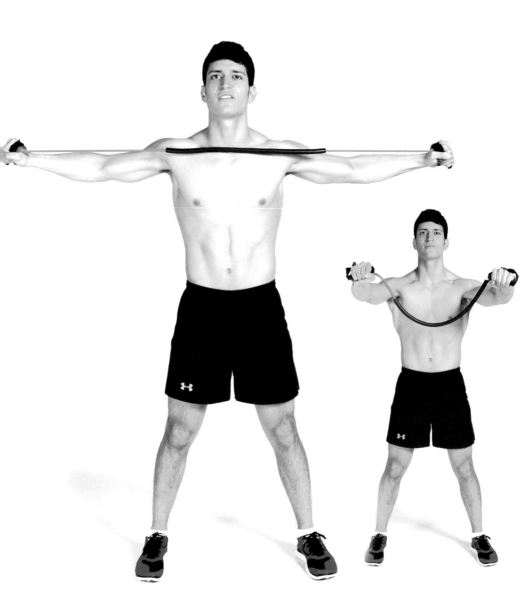

HOW TO DO IT

1 Stand with your feet shoulder-width apart, holding a band straight out in front of you. Your hands should also be shoulder-width apart.

2 Perform a fly motion, pulling the band across your chest and out to the sides, while keeping your palms facing down. Pause for a moment, then return to the starting position. Repeat 10–15 times.

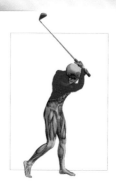

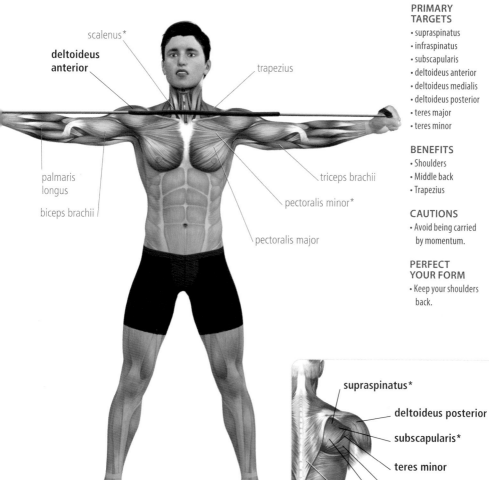

scalenus*

deltoideus anterior

trapezius

palmaris longus

biceps brachii

triceps brachii

pectoralis minor*

pectoralis major

PRIMARY TARGETS
- supraspinatus
- infraspinatus
- subscapularis
- deltoideus anterior
- deltoideus medialis
- deltoideus posterior
- teres major
- teres minor

BENEFITS
- Shoulders
- Middle back
- Trapezius

CAUTIONS
- Avoid being carried by momentum.

PERFECT YOUR FORM
- Keep your shoulders back.

supraspinatus*

deltoideus posterior

subscapularis*

teres minor

teres major

infraspinatus*

erector spinae*

ANNOTATION KEY

Black text indicates strengthening muscles
Gray text indicates stretching muscles
Italic text indicates tendons and ligaments
- - - - *indicates deep muscles

EXTERNAL ROTATION WITH BAND

BEGINNER

THE EXTERNAL ROTATION WITH BAND is a simple routine to increase power and strength in the shoulder muscles. It is also useful for boosting your triceps and forearms.

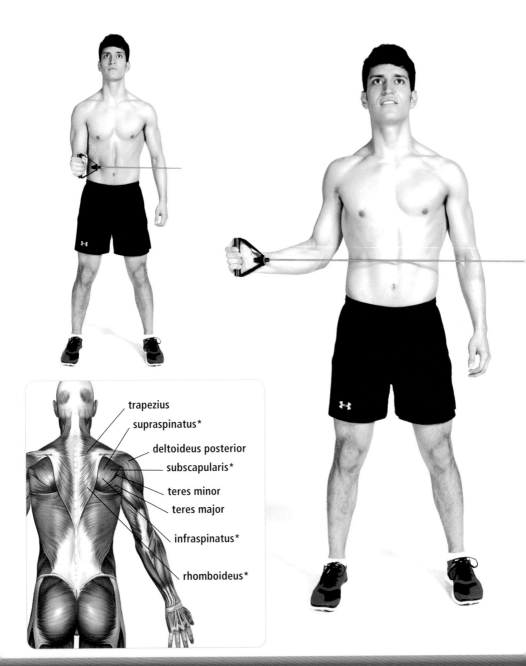

trapezius
supraspinatus*
deltoideus posterior
subscapularis*
teres minor
teres major
infraspinatus*
rhomboideus*

HOW TO DO IT

1 Fasten one end of a band around a post at elbow height. Grasp the other end with your right hand, keeping your upper arm pressed against your side and your forearm parallel to the ground.

2 Keeping your upper arm in position, move your forearm as far out to the side as you can before returning to the starting position. Complete 12–15 repetitions, then switch to the other arm.

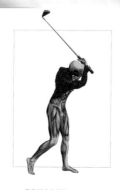

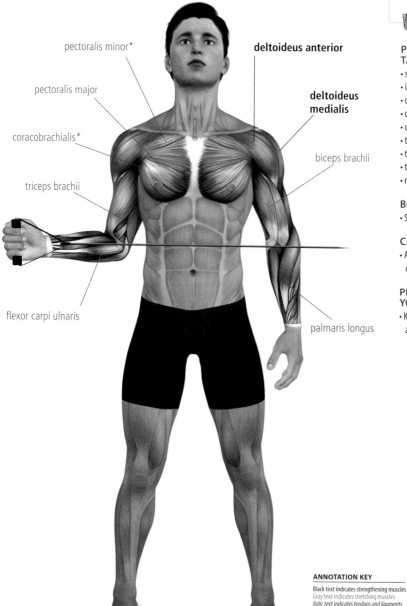

pectoralis minor*

pectoralis major

coracobrachialis*

triceps brachii

flexor carpi ulnaris

deltoideus anterior

deltoideus medialis

biceps brachii

palmaris longus

PRIMARY TARGETS
- supraspinatus
- infraspinatus
- deltoideus anterior
- deltoideus medialis
- deltoideus posterior
- teres major
- teres minor
- trapezius
- rhomboideus

BENEFITS
- Shoulders

CAUTIONS
- Avoid working at an excessively fast pace.

PERFECT YOUR FORM
- Keep your upper arm against your side.

ANNOTATION KEY

Black text indicates strengthening muscles
Gray text indicates stretching muscles
Italic text indicates tendons and ligaments
- - - - *indicates deep muscles

HEEL RAISE WITH OVERHEAD PRESS

BEGINNER

ALTHOUGH YOU CAN LIFT more weight with the Bench Press than with the Overhead Press, the Overhead Press has many benefits over the Bench Press, the main one being that it works your body as one piece. Your trunk and legs stabilize the weight while your shoulders, upper-chest and arms press the weight overhead.

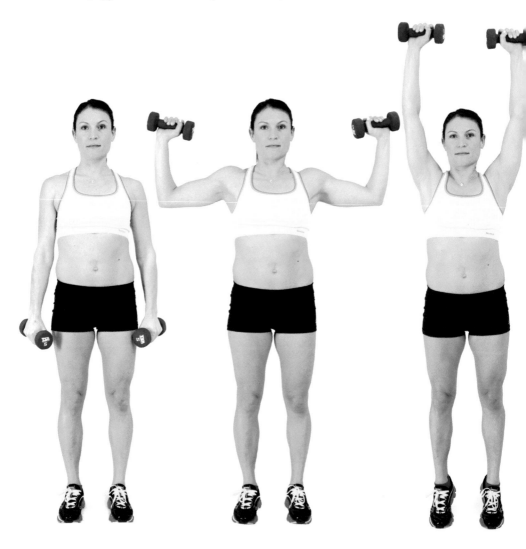

HOW TO DO IT

1 Stand with your feet hip-width apart and your arms at your sides, a dumbbell in each hand.

2 Raise your arms, bending your elbows and lifting until the dumbbells are at ear height.

3 Bring your weights overhead as you lift your heels off the floor to stand on your tiptoes. Balance for a few seconds, if desired.

4 Lower your heels to the floor and bring your arms back to starting position. Repeat, aiming for 15 repetitions with good form.

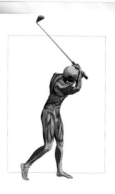

PRIMARY TARGETS
- gastrocnemius
- latissimus dorsi
- deltoideus anterior

BENEFITS
- Strengthens and tones shoulders and calves

CAUTIONS
- Tilting or twisting your torso.
- Hunching your shoulders.
- Arching your back or hunching forward.
- Holding your breath while in the lifted position.

PERFECT YOUR FORM
- Keep your torso facing forward.

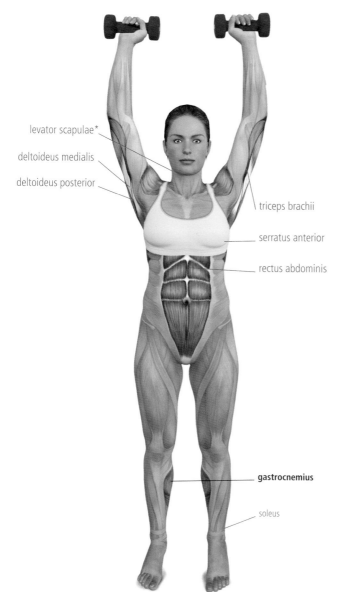

levator scapulae*

deltoideus medialis

deltoideus posterior

triceps brachii

serratus anterior

rectus abdominis

gastrocnemius

soleus

SQUAT AND ROW

ADVANCED

THE SQUAT AND ROW is an advanced full-body exercise. This is an excellent compound exercise that targets the glutes, quads, back and arms and would be suitable for any fitness level.

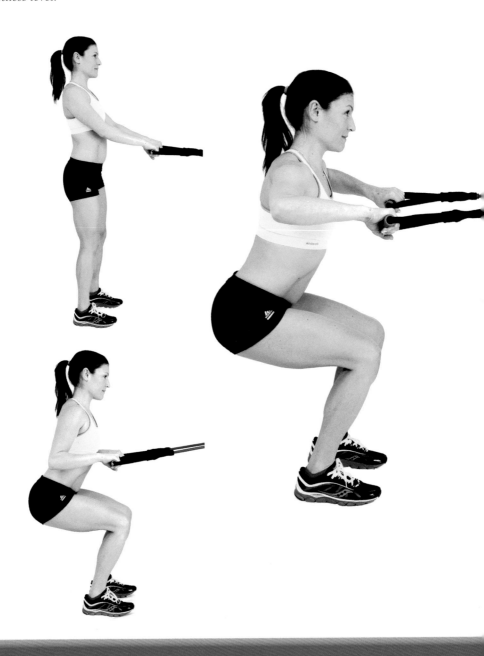

HOW TO DO IT

1 Stand upright, holding both ends of a resistance band in your hands. Your feet should be planted hip-width apart, your back neither arched nor slumped. Gaze forward.

2 In a smooth movement, begin to bend your knees. At the same time, bend your elbows as you pull both ends of the band in toward your body.

3 Keeping the rest of your body stable and your abdominal muscles engaged, use both hands to pull the band even further toward your body.

4 Smoothly return to starting position. Repeat, starting with 10 repetitions and building up to 20.

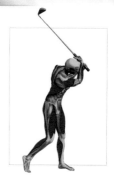

PRIMARY TARGETS
- gluteus maximus
- rectus femoris
- vastus lateralis
- vastus intermedius*
- vastus medialis
- biceps femoris
- semitendinosus
- semimembranosus
- latissimus dorsi
- pectoralis major

BENEFITS
- Strengthens and tones leg, gluteal and shoulder muscles
- Builds endurance

CAUTIONS
- Twisting your torso.
- Arching your back.
- Rushing through the movement.
- Twisting your neck to either side.
- Lowering your chin.

PERFECT YOUR FORM
- Keep both feet anchored to the ground.
- When bending, aim for your legs to form a right angle.
- Move slowly and with control.
- Keep your belly pulled inward.

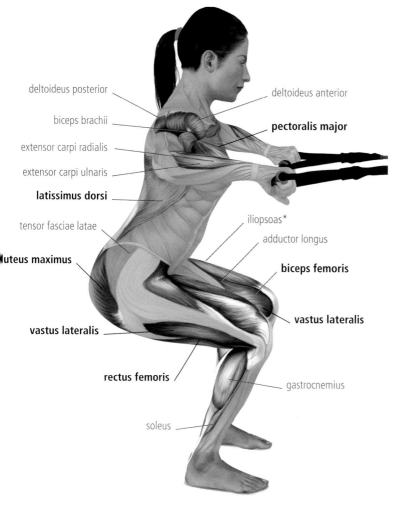

deltoideus posterior

biceps brachii

extensor carpi radialis

extensor carpi ulnaris

latissimus dorsi

tensor fasciae latae

Gluteus maximus

vastus lateralis

rectus femoris

soleus

deltoideus anterior

pectoralis major

iliopsoas*

adductor longus

biceps femoris

vastus lateralis

gastrocnemius

ANNOTATION KEY

Black text indicates strengthening muscles
Gray text indicates stretching muscles
Italic text indicates tendons and ligaments
- - - - *indicates deep muscles

REVERSE LUNGE WITH CHEST PRESS

INTERMEDIATE

THIS MOVE IS GOOD for those who are looking to work their upper body, specifically the chest and shoulders, and lower body at one time. It can be performed with cables or dumbbells—be sure to select a weight or resistance that you can control but will still add some form of a challenge to the exercise.

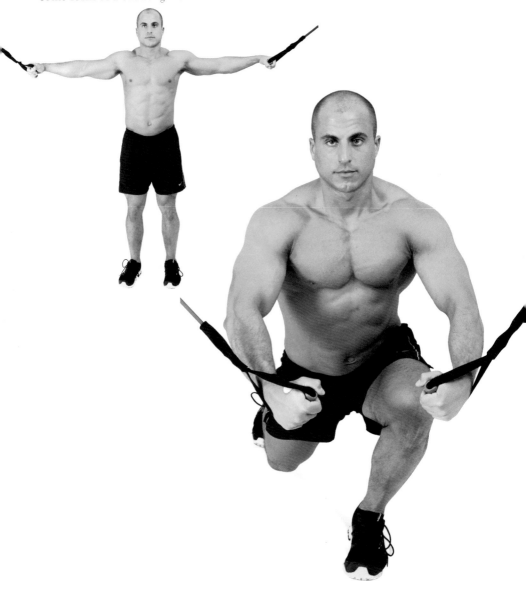

HOW TO DO IT

1 Stand upright with your feet roughly hip-width apart. Grasp the handle of one resistance band in each hand. Loop the other handles of both bands around weight machines or other stable objects to either side of you. Raise your arms to hold both bands perpendicular to your body, slightly taut.

2 Step your left leg behind you.

3 Bend both knees into a reverse lunge position. At the same time lower both arms, feeling resistance on the bands.

4 Gradually straighten your legs, and raise your arms to your sides to return to starting position.

5 Step your left leg forward, and repeat on the other side. Alternating, aim for 10 repetitions on each side.

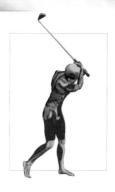

PRIMARY TARGETS
• rectus femoris
• vastus lateralis
• vastus intermedius*
• vastus medialis
• biceps femoris
• semitendinosus
• semimembranosus
• gluteus maximus
• pectoralis major

BENEFITS
• Strengthens and tones arms and chest muscles
• Improves coordination

CAUTIONS
• Avoid twisting your torso in either direction.
• Hunching your shoulders.

PERFECT YOUR FORM
• Keep your torso facing forward.

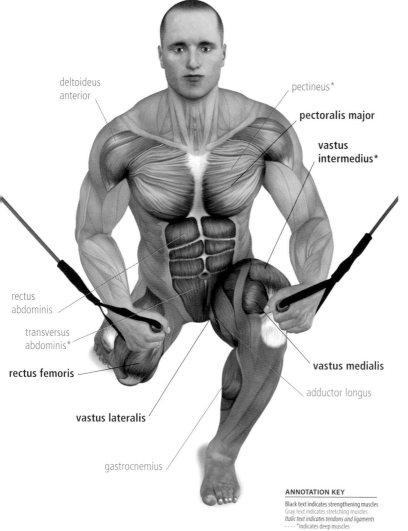

deltoideus anterior

pectineus*

pectoralis major

vastus intermedius*

rectus abdominis

transversus abdominis*

rectus femoris

vastus lateralis

gastrocnemius

vastus medialis

adductor longus

ANNOTATION KEY

Black text indicates strengthening muscles
Gray text indicates stretching muscles
Italic text indicates tendons and ligaments
---- *indicates deep muscles

CHIN-UP WITH HANGING LEG RAISE

ADVANCED

THIS IS AN AWESOME—and challenging—exercise to blast the upper back and the core at the same time with one movement. Perform hanging leg raises while holding the top position of a chin-up.

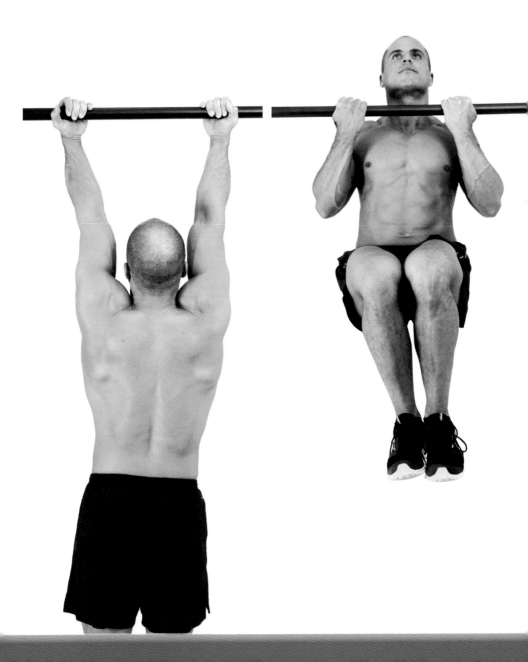

HOW TO DO IT

1 Begin hanging from a chin-up bar, gripping it firmly with both hands.

2 Use your arm muscles to lift yourself up, aiming to bring your chin over the bar.

3 With your abdominal muscles strongly engaged, raise your knees. Hold for as long as possible.

4 Slowly straighten your legs. Then, straighten your arms as you return to starting position.

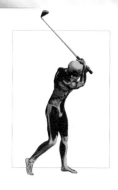

PRIMARY TARGETS
- latissimus dorsi
- rectus abdominis
- obliquus externus
- transversus abdominis*
- obliquus internus*
- serratus anterior
- triceps brachii

BENEFITS
- Strengthens arms and core

CAUTIONS
- Avoid moving in a jerky manner.

PERFECT YOUR FORM
- Engage your core muscles throughout this challenging exercise.

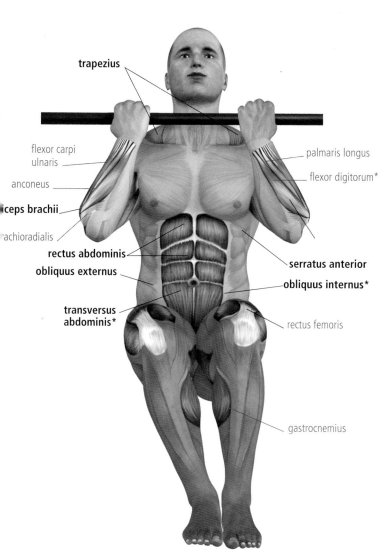

trapezius

flexor carpi ulnaris

anconeus

ceps brachii

achioradialis

rectus abdominis

obliquus externus

transversus abdominis*

palmaris longus

flexor digitorum*

serratus anterior

obliquus internus*

rectus femoris

gastrocnemius

ANNOTATION KEY

Black text indicates strengthening muscles
Gray text indicates stretching muscles
Italic text indicates tendons and ligaments
---- *indicates deep muscles

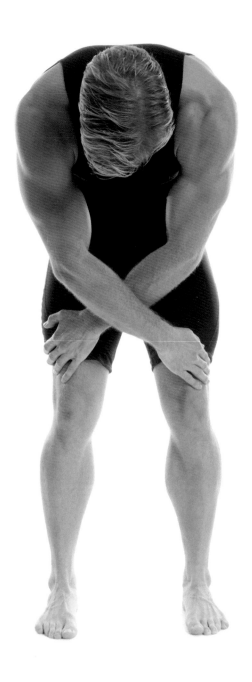

BACK

The golf swing isn't easy on our backs. Golfers are always dealing with stiff and achy backs, and all that twisting and bending can lead to back pain, or even injury. These back exercises are for golfers who want to avoid back pain and injury. Some focus on the lower back, others on the upper back. There are also a selection of stretching exercises that will not only loosen up your back to minimize pain but will also give you a greater backswing and follow-through range of motion, resulting in more power and distance with all your clubs.

NECK STRETCHES

STRETCH

NECK STRETCHES AND FLEXIBILITY EXERCISES can expand the range of motion and elasticity in the cervical spine area to help relieve stiffness and pain. Neck stretches should never be done to the point of pain or soreness.

DOWNWARD NECK TILT

HOW TO DO IT

1 Stand with your legs and feet parallel and shoulder-width apart. Bend your knees very slightly.

2 Tuck your pelvis about ¼ inch forward and stand tall, with your chest slightly lifted and shoulders pressed lightly downward and back, away from your ears.

3 Slowly tilt your head to the right, feeling the weight of your head shifting in this direction as you hold for 5 seconds.

4 Slowly return your head to the center, rest for 5 seconds, and repeat on the other side.

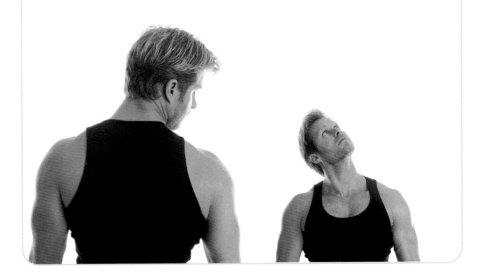

UPWARD NECK TILT

HOW TO DO IT

1 Clasp your hands behind your head, interlacing your fingers. Gently tilt your head forward, and hold for 5 seconds.

2 Slowly bring your head back up, rest for 5 seconds, and repeat.

MODIFICATION

To deepen this stretch, again place one hand on your head, and "reach for the keys" with the other.

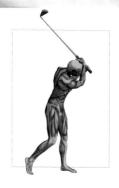

BACK-OF THE NECK STRETCH

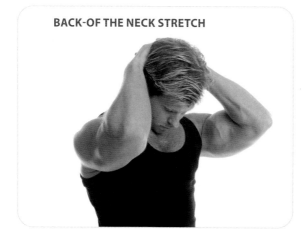

PRIMARY TARGETS
• sternocleidomastoideus
• splenius
• levator scapulae
• trapezius
• ligamentum interspinalis
• ligamentum capsular facet

BENEFITS
• Neck

CAUTIONS
• Avoid lifting or tensing your shoulders.

PERFECT YOUR FORM
• Breathe easily and normally during all of the stretches.

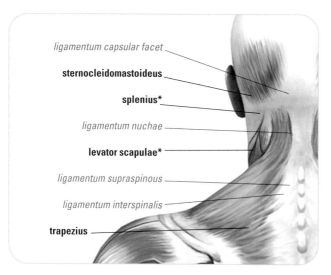

ligamentum capsular facet

sternocleidomastoideus

splenius*

ligamentum nuchae

levator scapulae*

ligamentum supraspinous

ligamentum interspinalis

trapezius

ANNOTATION KEY

Black text indicates strengthening muscles
Gray text indicates stretching muscles
Italic text indicates tendons and ligaments
- - - - *indicates deep muscles

STANDING BACK ROLL

STRETCH

THIS STRETCH PROMOTES FLEXIBILITY in the upper and middle back. Though the back is often overlooked as part of a warm-up or cooldown, stretching it will help reduce general muscle aches after an intense workout.

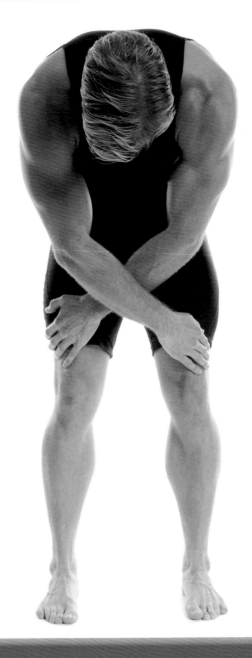

HOW TO DO IT

1 Lie on your back with both legs extended and your spine in an imprinted position so that your lower back touches the floor.

2 With your hands placed on your hamstrings just below the knee, extend and straighten your left leg upward.

3 Point both feet, and hold this postion for 15 to 30 seconds.

4 Switch legs, and repeat the stretch on the other side.

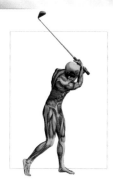

PRIMARY TARGETS

- extensor carpi radialis
- extensor carpi ulnaris
- extensor digiti minimi
- extensor digitorum
- extensor indicis
- extensor pollicis

BENEFITS

- Wrists
- Hands
- Forearms

CAUTIONS

- Avoid lifting or tensing your shoulders.

PERFECT YOUR FORM

- Be sure to press your thumb into the meaty part of your palm, attached to the thumb, intensifying the stretch in your forearm and wrist.

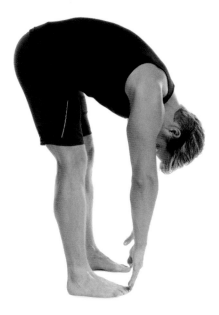

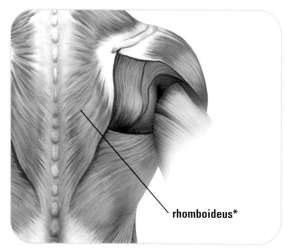

rhomboideus*

SCOOP RHOMBOIDS

STRETCH

THIS STRETCH PROMOTES flexibility in the upper and middle back. Though the back is often overlooked as part of a warm-up or cooldown, stretching it will help reduce general muscle aches after an intense workout.

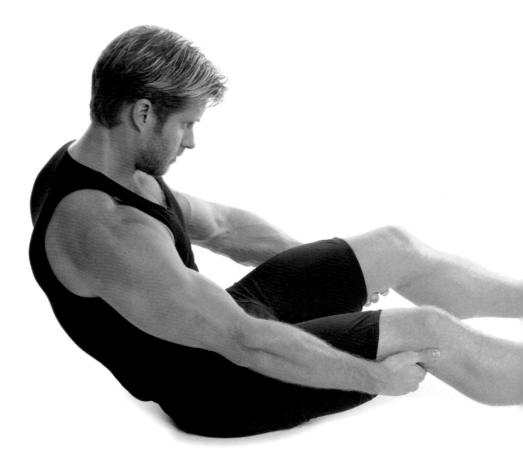

HOW TO DO IT

1 Sit on the floor and extend your legs in front of you in parallel position. Bend your knees slightly, keeping your heels on the floor.

2 Grasp beneath your hamstrings with your hands.

3 Keeping your chin down, round your upper back down as you lean back toward the floor. Hold for 10 to 15 seconds.

4 Slowly roll up to the starting position, and repeat if desired.

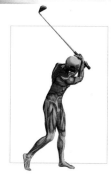

PRIMARY TARGETS
• Rhomboideus

BENEFITS
• Upper back

CAUTIONS
• Avoid holding your breath.

PERFECT YOUR FORM
• Exhale as you round your upper back and lean backward.

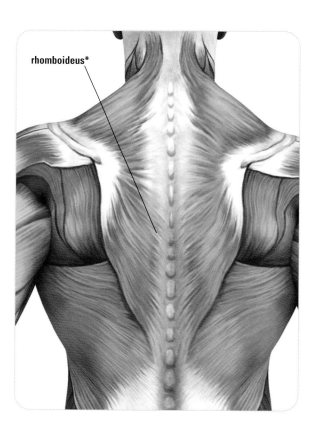

rhomboideus*

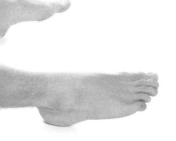

ANNOTATION KEY

Black text indicates strengthening muscles
Gray text indicates stretching muscles
Italic text indicates tendons and ligaments
- - - - *indicates deep muscles

LAT PULLDOWNS

BEGINNER

LAT PULLDOWNS focus on the latissimus dorsi, forearms and biceps, increasing strength and width in the back muscles. A wider grip makes for an easier routine as it reduces your range of motion, while a closer grip does the opposite and so makes it more of a challenge.

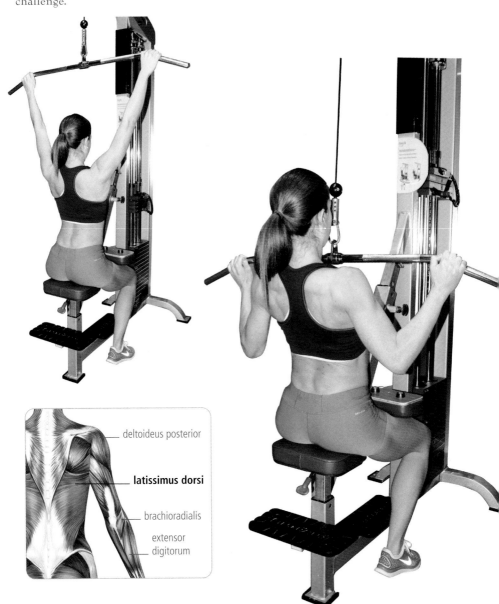

deltoideus posterior

latissimus dorsi

brachioradialis

extensor digitorum

HOW TO DO IT

1 Begin in a seated position at the pulldown machine. Grab the bar with an overhand grip that is slightly wider than shoulder-width.

2 Pull the bar down to the very top of your chest.

3 Fully extend your arms overhead using a controlled movement. Complete 8–10 repetitions.

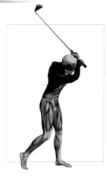

PRIMARY TARGETS
• latissimus dorsi

BENEFITS
• Forearms
• Biceps

CAUTIONS
• Avoid pulling the bar behind your neck.

PERFECT YOUR FORM
• Always sit up straight, maintaining a flat back.

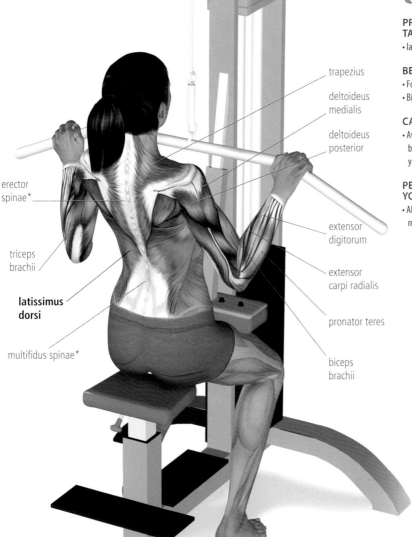

trapezius

deltoideus medialis

deltoideus posterior

erector spinae*

extensor digitorum

triceps brachii

extensor carpi radialis

latissimus dorsi

pronator teres

multifidus spinae*

biceps brachii

ANNOTATION KEY
Black text indicates strengthening muscles
Gray text indicates stretching muscles
Italic text indicates tendons and ligaments
- - - - *indicates deep muscles

ALTERNATING KETTLEBELL ROW

BEGINNER

THE ALTERNATING KETTLEBELL ROW builds strength in the middle back. It also benefits the biceps and latissimus dorsi. You can make the exercise less challenging by lifting with both arms at the same time, or more difficult by raising one leg off the floor.

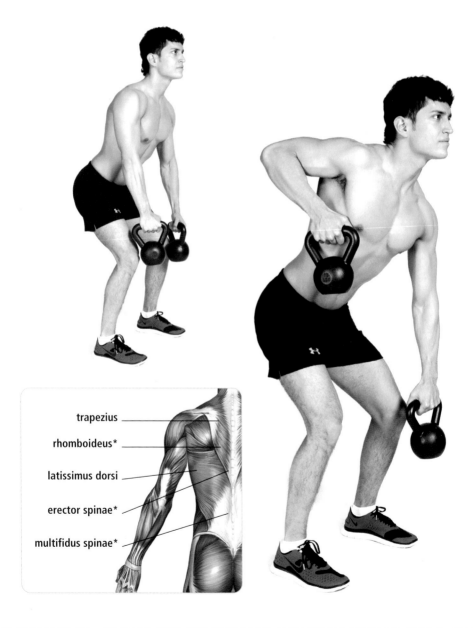

trapezius

rhomboideus*

latissimus dorsi

erector spinae*

multifidus spinae*

HOW TO DO IT

1 Stand upright with your feet shoulder-width apart. Hold a pair of kettlebells in front of you with an overhand grip. Bend forward slightly at the waist, maintaining a flat back.

2 Next, pull your right hand up, then lower it. Complete 8–10 repetitions per hand.

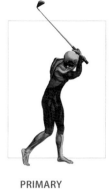

PRIMARY TARGETS

- trapezius
- rhomboideus
- latissimus dorsi
- erector spinae
- multifidus spinae

BENEFITS

- Middle back
- Biceps
- Latissimus dorsi

CAUTIONS

- Avoid rotating your core.

PERFECT YOUR FORM

- Maintain a flat back during the exercise.

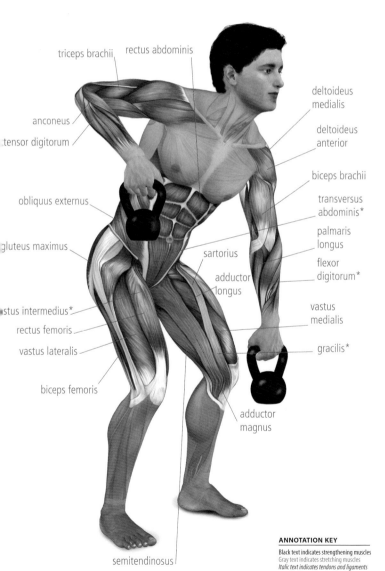

triceps brachii

rectus abdominis

anconeus

tensor digitorum

obliquus externus

gluteus maximus

stus intermedius*

rectus femoris

vastus lateralis

biceps femoris

semitendinosus

deltoideus medialis

deltoideus anterior

biceps brachii

transversus abdominis*

palmaris longus

flexor digitorum*

vastus medialis

gracilis*

sartorius

adductor longus

adductor magnus

ANNOTATION KEY

Black text indicates strengthening muscles
Gray text indicates stretching muscles
Italic text indicates tendons and ligaments
- - - - *indicates deep muscles

ALTERNATING RENEGADE ROW

ADVANCED

ANOTHER GREAT ROUTINE for the middle back, the Alternating Renegade Row also strengthens the abdominals, biceps, chest, latissimus dorsi and triceps.

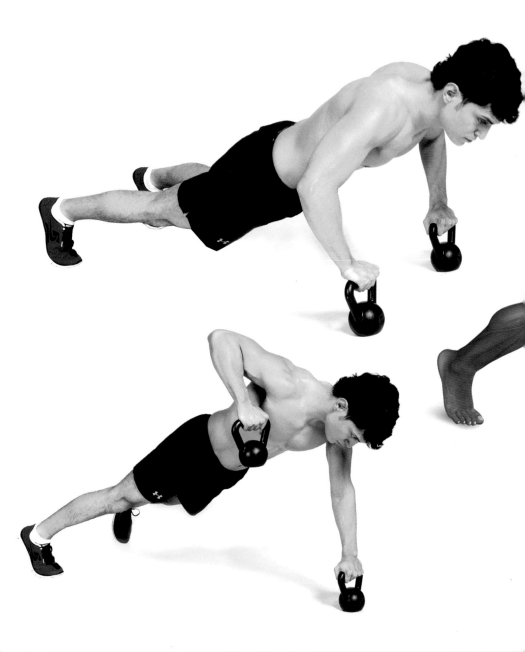

HOW TO DO IT

1 With a kettlebell in each hand, plant yourself on the floor in a push-up position.

2 While staying up on your toes and keeping your core stable and parallel to the floor, pull the kettlebell in your right hand up toward your chest while straightening the left arm and pushing that kettlebell into the floor.

3 Lower your right arm, then repeat the movement with the left. Complete 8–10 repetitions per arm.

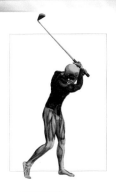

PRIMARY TARGETS
• trapezius
• rhomboideus
• latissimus dorsi
• erector spinae
• multifidus spinae

BENEFITS
• Middle back
• Abdominals
• Biceps
• Chest
• Triceps

CAUTIONS
• Avoid dropping or slamming the weight into the floor.

PERFECT YOUR FORM
• Keep your core stable and straight on.

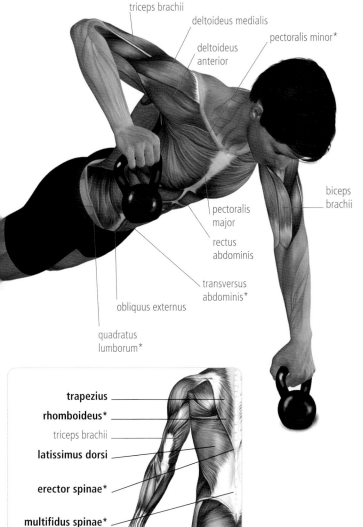

triceps brachii

deltoideus medialis

pectoralis minor*

deltoideus anterior

biceps brachii

pectoralis major

rectus abdominis

transversus abdominis*

obliquus externus

quadratus lumborum*

trapezius

rhomboideus*

triceps brachii

latissimus dorsi

erector spinae*

multifidus spinae*

ANNOTATION KEY

Black text indicates strengthening muscles
Gray text indicates stretching muscles
Italic text indicates tendons and ligaments
---- *indicates deep muscles

SWISS BALL HIP CROSSOVER

ADVANCED

THE SWISS BALL HIP CROSSOVER increases rotational strength of the midsection. The exercise targets the core, hips and lower back while also improving balance and stability.

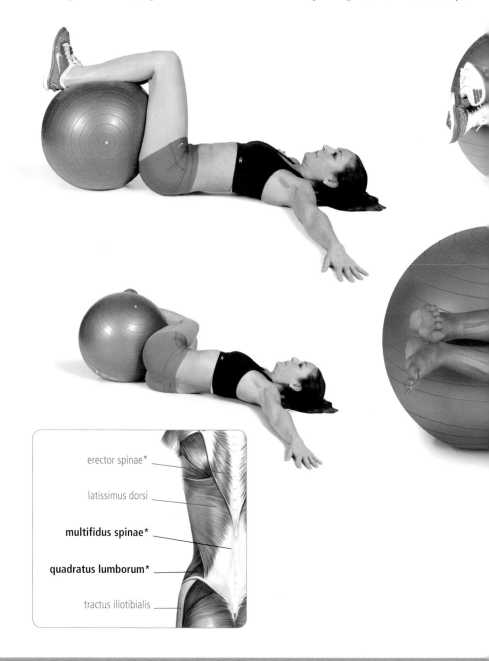

erector spinae*

latissimus dorsi

multifidus spinae*

quadratus lumborum*

tractus iliotibialis

HOW TO DO IT

1 Lie on your back with your arms stretched out to your sides. Place your legs on a Swiss ball, with your glutes close to it, bending your knees at 90 degrees.

2 Brace your abdominals, and lower your legs to the right side until they are as close to the floor as possible. Do not lift your shoulders off the floor.

3 Return to the starting position, then rotate your legs to the other side. Complete 15 repetitions per side.

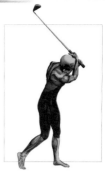

PRIMARY TARGETS
- multifidus spinae
- quadratus lumborum
- obliquus externus
- obliquus internus
- rectus abdominis

BENEFITS
- Lower back
- Obliques

CAUTIONS
- Avoid swinging your legs excessively.

PERFECT YOUR FORM
- Keep your core centred.

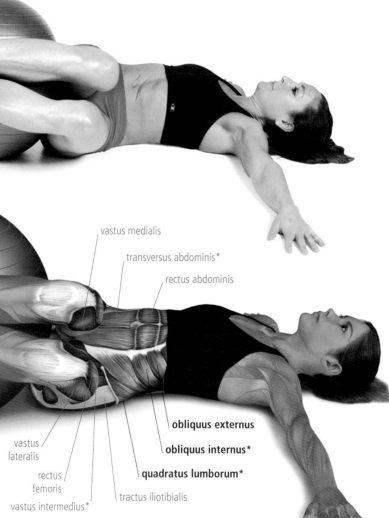

vastus medialis

transversus abdominis*

rectus abdominis

vastus lateralis

rectus femoris

vastus intermedius*

tractus iliotibialis

obliquus externus

obliquus internus*

quadratus lumborum*

ANNOTATION KEY

Black text indicates strengthening muscles
Gray text indicates stretching muscles
Italic text indicates tendons and ligaments
- - - - *indicates deep muscles

BARBELL POWER CLEAN

INTERMEDIATE

BARBELL POWER CLEANS are an explosive weightlifting exercise in which you lift a barbell from the floor to your shoulders in a continuous, powerful movement. The barbell power clean is a compound exercise movement, which means multiple muscle groups are utilized in the exercise—in this instance your glutes, deltoids, hamstrings, quads, core and upper back.

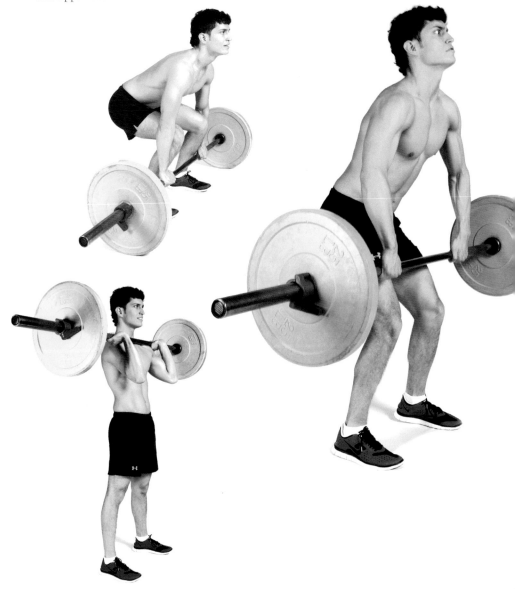

HOW TO DO IT

1 Stand in front of a barbell with your feet shoulder-width apart. Looking straight ahead, squat down and grab the barbell with a wide overhand grip. Your knees should be close to the bar.

2 Straighten your legs to return to a standing position. As you do so, flip the bar until it is nearly touching your upper chest.

3 From the upper chest, reverse your flip and return to the starting position. Complete 6–8 repetitions.

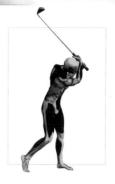

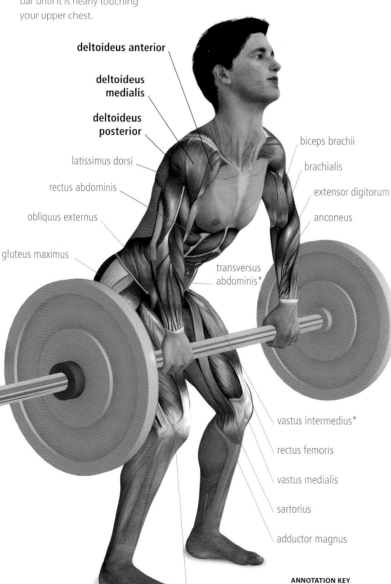

- deltoideus anterior
- deltoideus medialis
- deltoideus posterior
- latissimus dorsi
- rectus abdominis
- obliquus externus
- gluteus maximus
- biceps brachii
- brachialis
- extensor digitorum
- anconeus
- transversus abdominis*
- vastus intermedius*
- rectus femoris
- vastus medialis
- sartorius
- adductor magnus
- vastus lateralis

PRIMARY TARGETS
- deltoideus anterior
- deltoideus medialis
- deltoideus posterior
- trapezius
- infraspinatus
- supraspinatus
- teres major
- teres minor
- subscapularis

BENEFITS
- Deltoids
- Upper back
- Thighs
- Glutes
- Hamstrings
- Core

CAUTIONS
- Avoid overarching your back.

PERFECT YOUR FORM
- Be sure to use your legs to help with the movement.

ANNOTATION KEY
Black text indicates strengthening muscles
Gray text indicates stretching muscles
Italic text indicates tendons and ligaments
- - - - *indicates deep muscles

FULL BODY ROLL

INTERMEDIATE

THIS EXERCISE IS an excellent way to stretch the back of the legs, groin, hips and back. Lying on your back and stretching in this movement is an effective way to get into tight spaces without compromising your back.

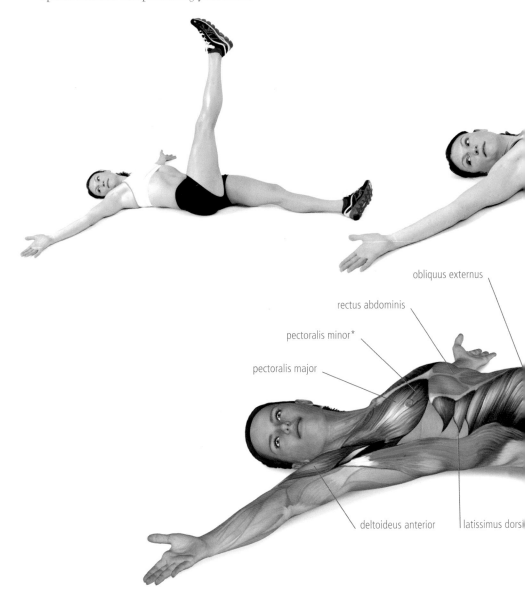

obliquus externus

rectus abdominis

pectoralis minor*

pectoralis major

deltoideus anterior

latissimus dorsi

HOW TO DO IT

1 Lie on your back, with your arms extended at your sides and your legs extended on the floor.

2 Raise your right leg so that it is perpendicular to the floor.

3 Lower your right leg toward the floor and then use your abdominal muscles and arms to roll to the left until you are face-down.

4 Straighten your arms, lifting your upper torso off the ground. Your legs should be extended behind you.

5 Roll onto your back, legs and arms extended in starting position. Then, raise your left leg and repeat the roll in the other direction. Repeat, alternating sides for 8 repetitions.

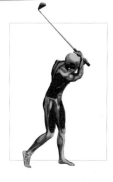

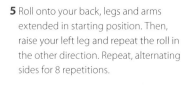

PRIMARY TARGETS
• vastus lateralis
• vastus intermedius*
• vastus medialis
• rectus femoris
• iliopsoas*
• biceps femoris
• semitendinosus
• semimembranosus
• gluteus maximus
• gluteus medius*
• gluteus minimus*

BENEFITS
• Tones cores muscles, especially obliques

CAUTIONS
• Avoid rushing through the movement.

PERFECT YOUR FORM
• Keep your abdominal muscles, especially your obliques, engaged as you roll.

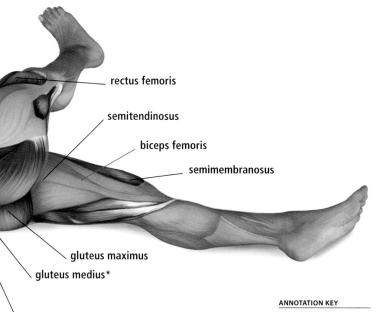

rectus femoris

semitendinosus

biceps femoris

semimembranosus

gluteus maximus

gluteus medius*

gluteus minimus*

ANNOTATION KEY

Black text indicates strengthening muscles
Gray text indicates stretching muscles
Italic text indicates tendons and ligaments
- - - - *indicates deep muscles

BACK ROLL

STRETCH

THE IDEA OF THIS exercise is to stretch your back and to pinpoint your sore muscles with a form of self massage. It shouldn't hurt, but when you find a tight ball of muscle that needs to loosen up, you'll definitely feel it!

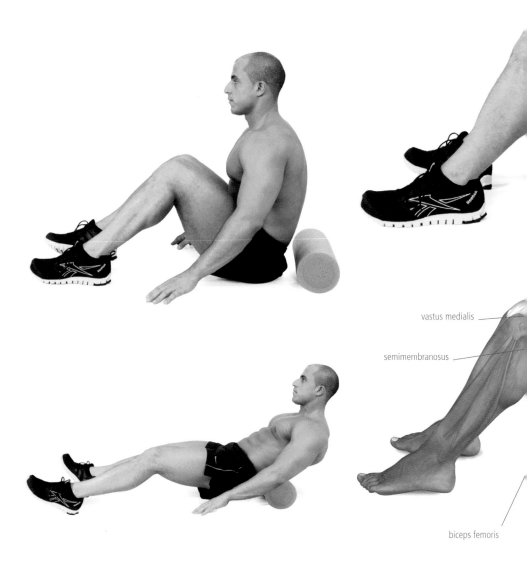

vastus medialis

semimembranosus

biceps femoris

HOW TO DO IT

1 Sit with your legs bent, extended in front of you, and your arms at your sides, palms on the floor. Position the foam roller behind you.

2 Extend your legs and lean back, engaging your core muscles as you rest your lower back on the roller.

3 Gradually roll forward until the roller is beneath your upper back.

4 Roll back to starting position. Repeat, completing 5 repetitions. Then, complete 5 more if desired.

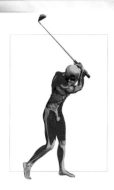

PRIMARY TARGETS
• latissimus dorsi
• rhomboideus*

BENEFITS
• Relieves soreness throughout back
• Improves range of motion

CAUTIONS
• Avoid arching your back.

PERFECT YOUR FORM
• Move smoothly and with control.
• Use your arms, legs and abs to drive the movement.

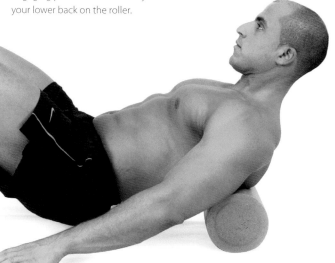

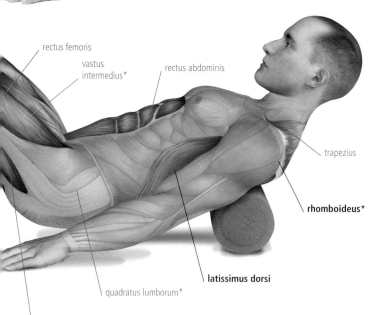

rectus femoris

vastus intermedius*

rectus abdominis

trapezius

rhomboideus*

latissimus dorsi

quadratus lumborum*

semitendinosus

ANNOTATION KEY
Black text indicates strengthening muscles
Gray text indicates stretching muscles
Italic text indicates tendons and ligaments
- - - - *indicates deep muscles

QUADRUPED LEG LIFT

BEGINNER

THIS EXERCISE STRENGTHENS the posterior core. The opposite arm and leg lift requires good rotational stability of the core to maintain proper form. This exercise can also enhance body awareness—placing a stick or tennis ball on the lower back gives extra feedback about the alignment of the spine.

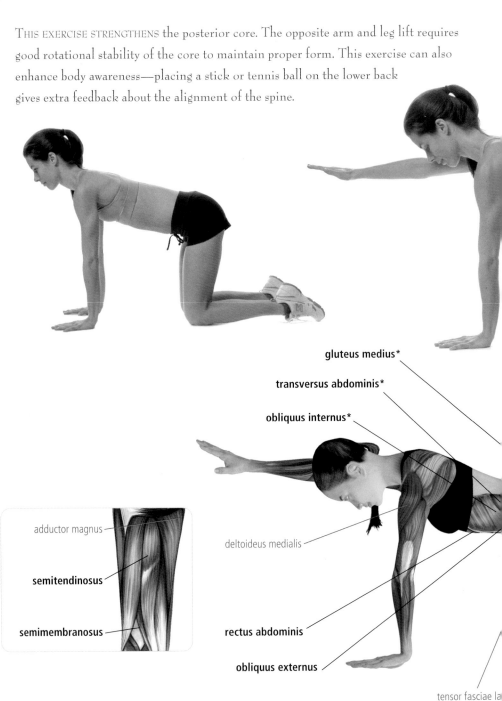

gluteus medius*

transversus abdominis*

obliquus internus*

adductor magnus

semitendinosus

semimembranosus

deltoideus medialis

rectus abdominis

obliquus externus

tensor fasciae la

HOW TO DO IT

1 Kneeling on all fours, connect with your abdominals by drawing your navel up toward your spine.

2 Slowly raise your right arm and extend your left leg, all while keeping your torso still. Extend your arm and leg until they are both parallel to the floor, creating one long line with your body. Do not allow your pelvis to bend or rotate.

3 Bring your arm and leg back into the starting position.

4 Repeat sequence on the other side, alternating sides six times.

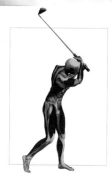

PRIMARY TARGETS

- rectus abdominis
- transversus abdominis
- obliquus internus
- obliquus externus
- gluteus maximus
- gluteus minimus
- gluteus medius
- biceps femoris
- semitendinosus
- semimembranosus

BENEFITS

- Abdominals
- Pelvic stabilisers
- Hip extensors
- Obliques

CAUTIONS

- Avoid tilting your pelvis during the movement – slide your leg along the surface of the floor before lifting.
- Allowing your back to sink into an arched position.

PERFECT YOUR FORM

- Keep your movement slow and steady to decrease pelvic rotation.
- Engage your abs by drawing your navel toward your spine.
- Press your shoulder blades down and back.

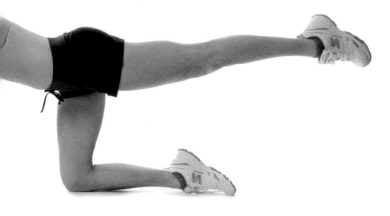

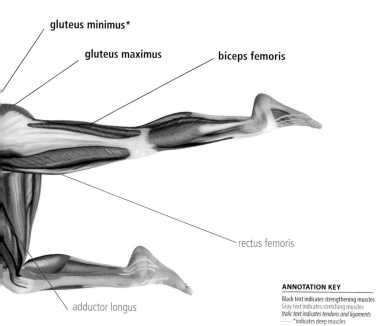

gluteus minimus*

gluteus maximus

biceps femoris

rectus femoris

adductor longus

ANNOTATION KEY

Black text indicates strengthening muscles
Gray text indicates stretching muscles
Italic text indicates tendons and ligaments
- - - - *indicates deep muscles

SWISS BALL EXTENSION

INTERMEDIATE

USING A BALL for back extensions creates an increased range of motion compared with what you get on the floor—and you'll also have a balance challenge since the ball is unstable. You may want to prop your feet against the wall to get more leverage.

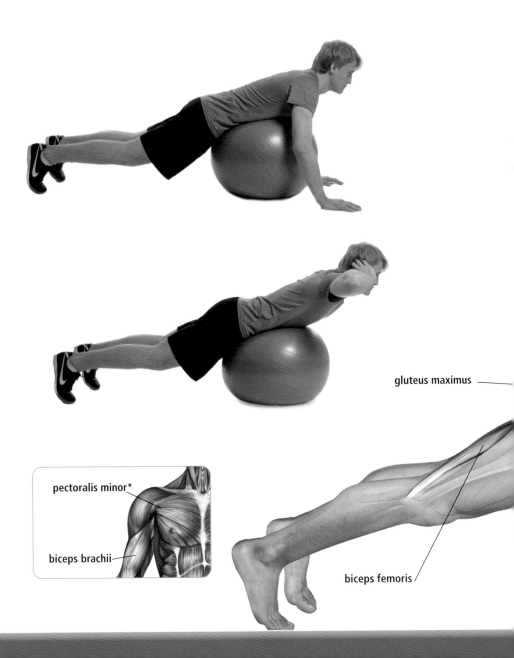

gluteus maximus

pectoralis minor*

biceps brachii

biceps femoris

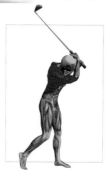

HOW TO DO IT

1 Lie prone over a Swiss ball, with your upper chest and head hanging off the edge of the ball.

2 Firmly plant your feet to stabilise yourself over the ball, and place your hands on either side of your head.

3 With arms bent and elbows out, raise your upper body off the ball.

4 Slowly and carefully lower your body to the starting position. Repeat ten times.

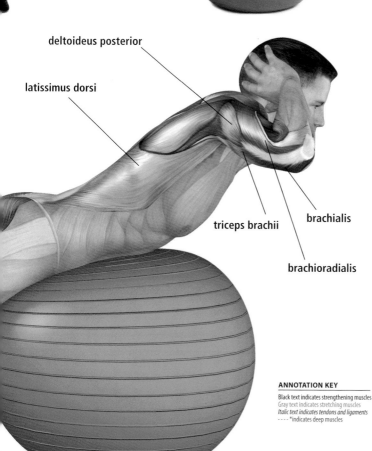

deltoideus posterior

latissimus dorsi

triceps brachii

brachialis

brachioradialis

PRIMARY TARGETS

- eerector spinae
- gluteus maximus
- biceps femoris
- semitendinosus
- semimembranosus
- adductor magnus
- latissimus dorsi
- teres major
- triceps brachii
- deltoideus posterior
- brachialis
- brachioradialis
- biceps brachii
- trapezius
- pectoralis minor
- rhomboideus
- multifidus spinae

BENEFITS
- Middle back
- Lower back

CAUTIONS
- Avoid elevating your shoulders.

PERFECT YOUR FORM
- Engage your glutes and thighs throughout the exercise.

ANNOTATION KEY
Black text indicates strengthening muscles
Gray text indicates stretching muscles
Italic text indicates tendons and ligaments
- - - - *indicates deep muscles

CLEAN AND LIFT

INTERMEDIATE

THE CLASSIC CLEAN AND LIFT boosts power and mass in the shoulders and upper back, especially the deltoids and triceps. It also benefits the thighs, glutes, hamstrings and core. Vary the difficulty levels by using dumbbells instead of a barbell, or a very light bar.

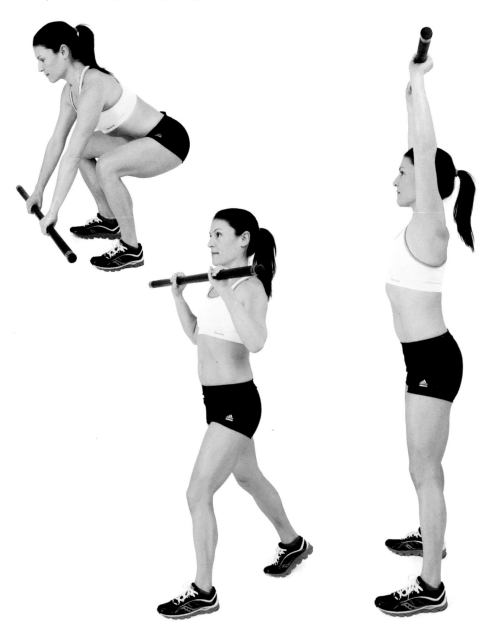

HOW TO DO IT

1 Begin in a high squatting position so that your upper legs are parallel with the floor. Hold the body bar in front of you, arms straight.

2 Using the muscles in your legs as well as your abdominals, rise to stand as you bend your arms to bring the bar to shoulder height. If you choose, extend one foot in front of the other.

3 Move your feet to parallel position, hip-width or wider apart, and bring the body bar above your head. Hold for several seconds.

4 Switch legs, and repeat on the stretch on the other side.

5 Repeat the lift overhead and the controlled lowering, aiming for 10 repetitions.

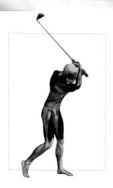

PRIMARY TARGETS
- latissimus dorsi
- trapezius
- deltoideus anterior
- deltoideus posterior
- deltoideus medialis
- triceps brachii
- serratus anterior
- supraspinatus*

BENEFITS
- Strengthens and tones whole body

CAUTIONS
- Avoid hunching your shoulders.
- Letting your abdominals bulge outward.
- Distorting the S-curve of your spine by arching your back or hunching forward.
- Rushing through the movement.

PERFECT YOUR FORM
- While you raise the bar overhead, keep your abdominals strongly engaged.

levator scapulae*

triceps brachii

deltoideus anterior

deltoideus posterior

deltoideus medialis

supraspinatus*

erector spinae*

serratus anterior

latissimus dorsi

rectus abdominis

transversus abdominis*

rectus femoris

vastus lateralis

ANNOTATION KEY
Black text indicates strengthening muscles
Gray text indicates stretching muscles
Italic text indicates tendons and ligaments
- - - - *indicates deep muscles

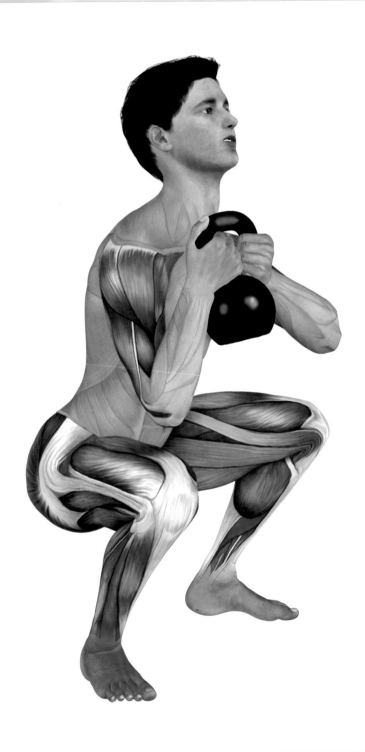

LEGS

We all know that our legs are important to our overall fitness, and especially so in the game of golf. They are important for many reasons, primarily stability, balance and power. Strengthening your legs will not only provide your swing with a strong base, but it will also help provide balance. Stronger legs will also help develop a more powerful golf swing through weight shifting. Your ankles will be one of the most important areas to target with exercise, allowing you to properly weight shift during the golf swing. Strengthening and improving the endurance of your quadriceps is key because you will be repetitively standing with your knees bent with each golf swing. The hamstrings come in to play when weight shifting and developing power when hitting through the ball.

CALF STRETCH

BEGINNER

PERFORM A FEW of these stretches during your cardiovascular workout—this will help relieve calf tightness and stress throughout your workout. With this exercise, avoid focusing downward—this might take the necessary weight off the front foot and onto the back leg, greatly decreasing the intensity of the stretch.

CALF HEEL DROP

HOW TO DO IT

1 Stand on a step, a raise or a stair with your legs and feet parallel and shoulder-width apart. Bend your knees very slightly and tuck your pelvis slightly forward, lift your chest and press your shoulders downward and back.

2 Position your left foot slightly in front of your right, and place the ball of your right foot on the edge of the step.

3 Drop your right heel down while controlling the amount of weight on the right leg to increase or decrease the intensity of the stretch in the right calf.

4 Release, switch feet and repeat on the other side.

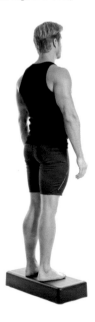

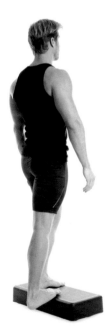

TOE-UP CALF STRETCH

HOW TO DO IT

1 Stand with your legs and feet parallel and shoulder-width apart. Bend your knees very slightly and tuck your pelvis slightly forward, lift your chest and press your shoulders downward and back.

2 Position the ball of your right foot on a step or against a wall.

3 With your knees straight, bring your hips forward.

4 Release, switch feet and repeat on the other side.

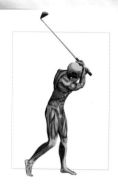

PRIMARY TARGETS
• gastrocnemius
• soleus
• tendo calcaneus

BENEFITS
• relieves tightness in the calves and muscles

CAUTIONS
• Avoid bouncing to achieve a greater stretch—all of your movements should be performed slowly and carefully.

PERFECT YOUR FORM
• Engage each head of your calf muscles by gently and slowly rolling from your big toe to your small toe and back again, shifting your body weight over your toes as you go.

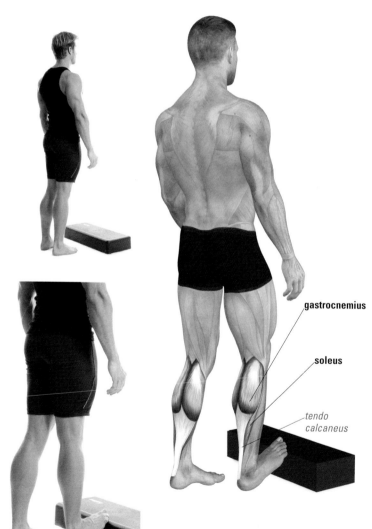

gastrocnemius

soleus

tendo calcaneus

ANNOTATION KEY
Black text indicates strengthening muscles
Gray text indicates stretching muscles
Italic text indicates tendons and ligaments
- - - - *indicates deep muscles

SIDE-LYING KNEE BEND

STRETCH

THIS EXERCISE TARGETS your quadriceps. Place a towel under your lower hip if it feels uncomfortable to rest directly on the floor. Avoid stretching further than feels comfortable.

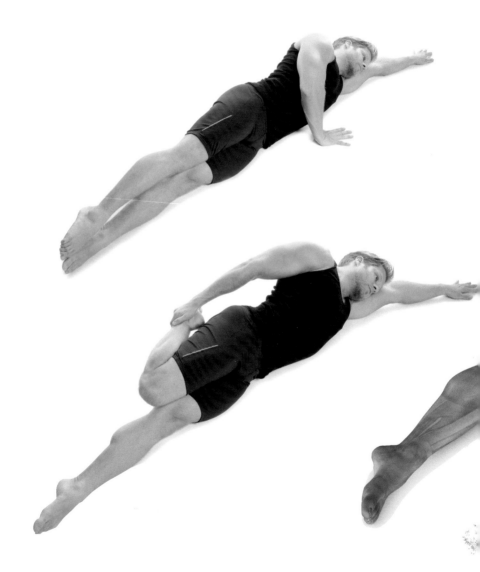

HOW TO DO IT

1 Lie on your left side, with your legs extended together in line with your body. Extend your left arm, and rest your head on your upper arm.

2 Bend your right knee and grasp the ankle with your right hand.

3 Pull your ankle in toward your buttocks as you stretch.

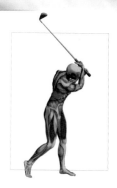

EXPERT'S TIP

Place a towel under your bottom hip if it feels uncomfortable to rest directly on the floor.

PRIMARY TARGETS

- rectus femoris
- vastus lateralis
- vastus intermedius
- vastus medialis

BENEFITS

- Quadriceps

CAUTIONS

- Avoid leaning back onto your gluteal muscles.

PERFECT YOUR FORM

- Keep your knees together, one on top of the other.
- Tuck your pelvis slightly forward and lift your chest to engage and stretch your core.
- Keep your foot pointed and parallel with your leg.

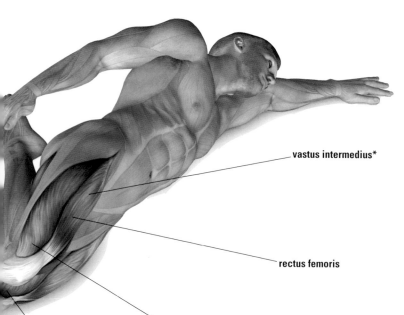

vastus intermedius*

rectus femoris

vastus lateralis

vastus medialis

ANNOTATION KEY

Black text indicates strengthening muscles
Gray text indicates stretching muscles
Italic text indicates tendons and ligaments
- - - - *indicates deep muscles

INTERNAL HIP ROTATOR STRETCH

INTERMEDIATE

THIS STRETCH IS NOT ABOUT BIG MOVES—you should internally rotate your hip no more than five inches as you stretch. Be sure to utilize a slow movement in both directions.

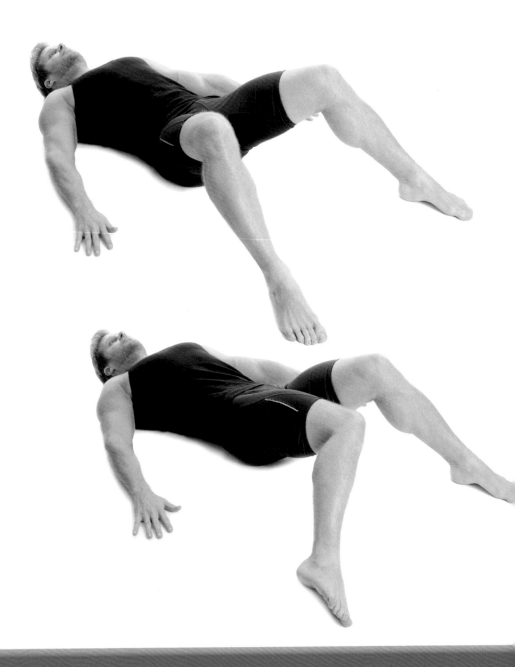

HOW TO DO IT

1 Lie on your back with your arms extended at your sides.

2 Bend your knees, planting your feet generously outside of shoulder-width.

3 Keeping the rest of your body still, rotate your right hip inward, bringing your knee toward the floor.

4 Slowly return to the starting position, and repeat with the opposite leg.

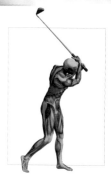

PRIMARY TARGETS
• gluteus medius
• gluteus minimus
• tensor fasciae latae

BENEFITS
• Hip rotators

CAUTIONS
• Avoid lifting your lower back and glutes.

PERFECT YOUR FORM
• Keep your abdominals tight and rest your hands on the floor to support your lower back.

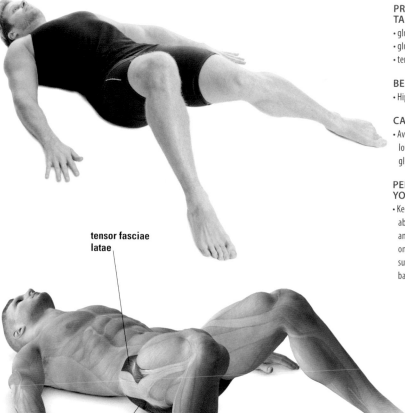

tensor fasciae latae

gluteus minimus*

gluteus medius*

ANNOTATION KEY
Black text indicates strengthening muscles
Gray text indicates stretching muscles
Italic text indicates tendons and ligaments
- - - - *indicates deep muscles

FROG STRADDLE

STRETCH

You can modify the Frog Straddle by moving your forearms forward and leaning into them. Try to keep both your pelvis and your heels on the floor as you stretch.

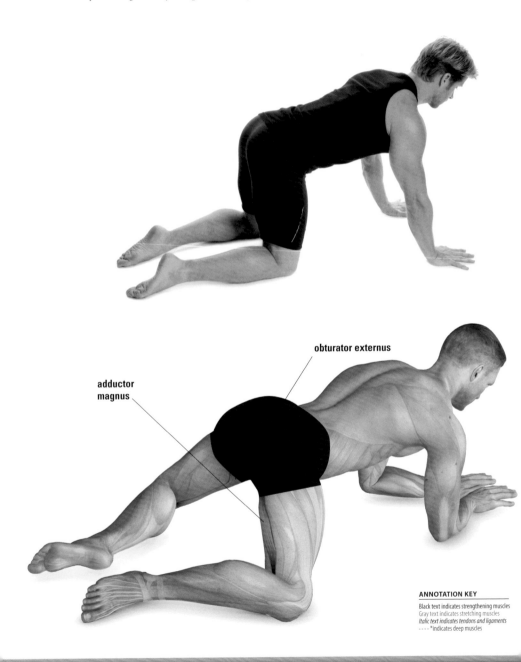

obturator externus

adductor magnus

ANNOTATION KEY

Black text indicates strengthening muscles
Gray text indicates stretching muscles
Italic text indicates tendons and ligaments
---- *indicates deep muscles

HOW TO DO IT

1 Kneel on all fours.

2 Bend your elbows and shift your weight forward so that you are leaning onto your elbows and forearms.

3 Spread your knees apart, drawing your feet in slightly and putting some weight on them to take pressure off your kneecaps. Make sure that there is very little weight resting on your knees.

4 Lower your legs and buttocks down to the floor and bring the soles of your feet together to deepen the stretch.

5 To safely come out of this stretch, bring your weight forward until you can extend your legs long behind you and you are lying on your stomach.

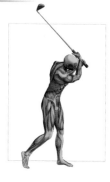

PRIMARY TARGETS
- adductor longus
- adductor magnus
- adductor brevis
- gracilis
- pectineus
- obturator externus

BENEFITS
- Inner thighs
- Hip adductors

CAUTIONS
- Avoid placing too much of your weight on your kneecaps.
- Allowing your lower back to sink.

PERFECT YOUR FORM
- Stretch until you reach a point of challenge without feeling pain.

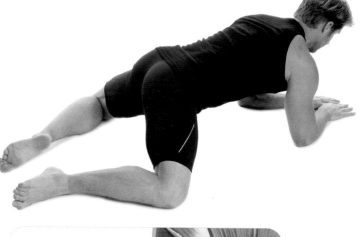

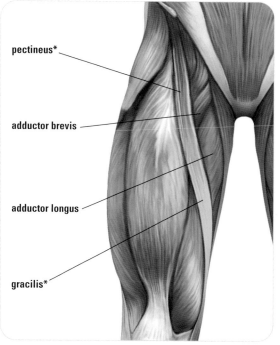

pectineus*

adductor brevis

adductor longus

gracilis*

UNILATERAL SEATED FORWARD BEND

INTERMEDIATE

THIS BEGINNER FORWARD BEND stretches the back of one leg at a time, making the exercise a little easier than a full forward bend with both legs in front. Keep the extended leg active, and focus on breathing in this movement.

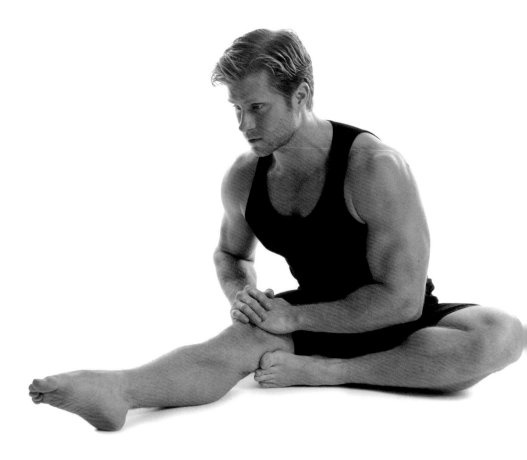

HOW TO DO IT

1 Sit on the floor, sitting up as straight as possible, with your legs extended in front of you in parallel position.

2 Bend your left leg until it is turned out, with the bottom of your left foot resting at your right inner thigh just above the kneecap. Rest your hands on your knee.

3 Bend from your waist and lean forward over your right leg. Place your forearms above your right kneecap.

4 Switch legs, and repeat on the stretch on the other side.

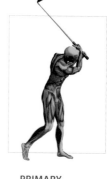

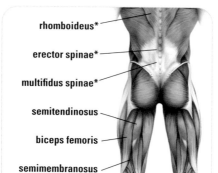

rhomboideus*

erector spinae*

multifidus spinae*

semitendinosus

biceps femoris

semimembranosus

PRIMARY TARGETS
- biceps femoris
- semitendinosus
- semimembranosus
- multifidus spinae
- erector spinae
- gastrocnemius
- soleus
- rhomboideus

BENEFITS
- Hamstrings

CAUTIONS
- Avoid straining your back—if yours is tight, try performing this stretch with a couch behind you.
- Be sure to position your lower back as close to the couch as possible.

PERFECT YOUR FORM
- Drop your head to benefit your rhomboids, and for a more intense overall stretch.

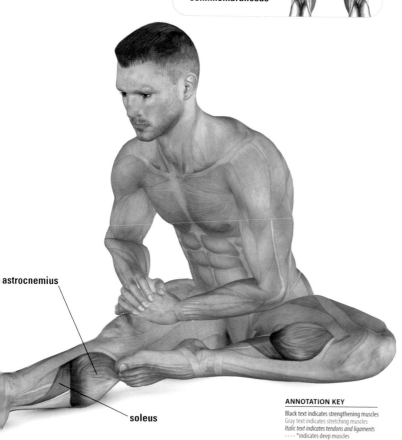

astrocnemius

soleus

ANNOTATION KEY

Black text indicates strengthening muscles
Gray text indicates stretching muscles
Italic text indicates tendons and ligaments
- - - - *indicates deep muscles

UNILATERAL LEG STRETCHES

STRETCH

PERFORM BOTH OF the Unilateral Leg Stretches followed by the Hip Extension and Flexion (Page 126), as a smooth sequence on one side before switching to the other and performing the sequence of exercises on the other side.

UNILATERAL KNEE-TO-CHEST STRETCH

HOW TO DO IT

1 Lie on your back, and bend your right knee in toward your chest.

2 Placing your hands on your right hamstrings, gently hug your knee closer to your chest as you stretch.

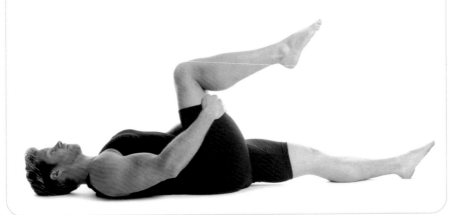

EXPERT'S TIP

Perform both of the Unilateral Leg Stretches followed by the Hip Adductor Stretch (see pages 198–199), as a smooth sequence on one side before switching to the other and performing all three stretches on the opposite side.

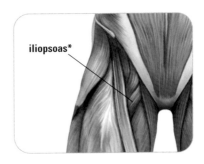

iliopsoas*

ANNOTATION KEY

Black text indicates strengthening muscles
Gray text indicates stretching muscles
Italic text indicates tendons and ligaments
---- *indicates deep muscles

UNILATERAL LEG RAISE

HOW TO DO IT

1 With your hands placed on your hamstrings just below the knee, extend and straighten your right leg toward the ceiling.

2 Point both feet.

3 Switch your hand position, right hand on your right calf muscle, left hand on your hamstring. Gently bring your thigh toward your chest, increasing the intensity of the stretch.

4 Prepare to move into the Hip Adductor Stretch (see pages 198–199).

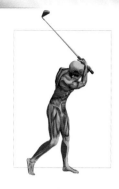

PRIMARY TARGETS
- erector spinae
- gluteus maximus
- gluteus medius
- gluteus minimus
- biceps femoris
- semitendinosus
- semimembranosus
- iliopsoas
- gastrocnemius
- soleus

BENEFITS
- Lower back
- Groin muscles
- Gluteal region
- Hamstrings

CAUTIONS
- Avoid lifting your head or upper back.
- Holding your breath.

PERFECT YOUR FORM
- Keep your lower back on the floor—tucking your pelvis just ¼ inch will help keep your back grounded.

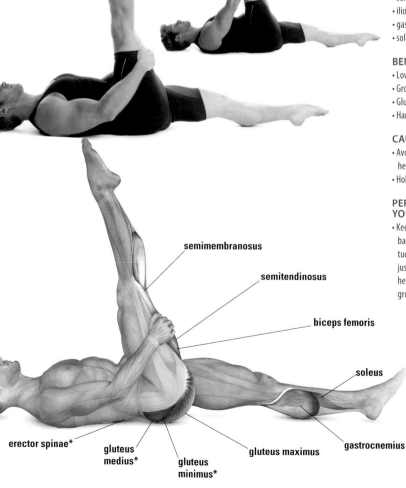

semimembranosus

semitendinosus

biceps femoris

soleus

gastrocnemius

erector spinae*

gluteus medius*

gluteus minimus*

gluteus maximus

BILATERAL SEATED FORWARD BEND

STRETCH

Seated Forward Bend is a basic yet challenging exercise that stretches the hamstrings, spine and lower back. Don't tense your jaw or clench your teeth while performing this stretch. Relaxing your mouth will help you breathe evenly.

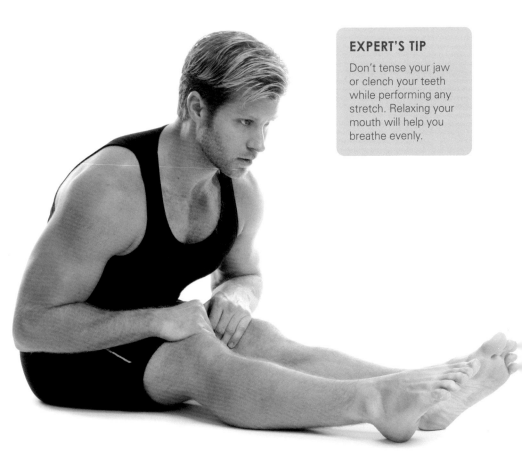

EXPERT'S TIP

Don't tense your jaw or clench your teeth while performing any stretch. Relaxing your mouth will help you breathe evenly.

HOW TO DO IT

1 Sit on the floor, sitting up as straight as possible with your back flattened and your legs extended in front of you in parallel position. Your feet should be relaxed and flexed slightly.

2 Lean forward, lowering your abdominals over your thighs, forearms resting above your kneecaps as you stretch.

3 Slowly roll up, and repeat if desired.

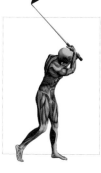

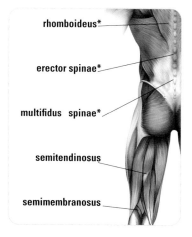

rhomboideus*

erector spinae*

multifidus   spinae*

semitendinosus

semimembranosus

ANNOTATION KEY
Black text indicates strengthening muscles
Gray text indicates stretching muscles
Italic text indicates tendons and ligaments
- - - - *indicates deep muscles

PRIMARY TARGETS
- biceps femoris
- semitendinosus
- semimembranosus
- multifidus spinae
- erector spinae
- gastrocnemius
- soleus
- rhomboideus

BENEFITS
- Hamstrings

CAUTIONS
- Avoid holding your breath.

PERFECT YOUR FORM
- Bend at the hips and keep your spine fairly straight as you stretch.
- Extend your torso as far forward over your legs as possible.

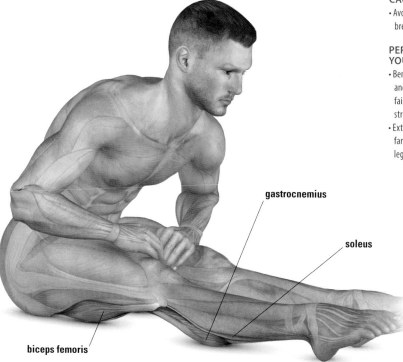

gastrocnemius

soleus

biceps femoris

GASTROCNEMIUS STRETCH

STRETCH

THE GASTROCNEMIUS MUSCLES attach to the leg below the knee, and when you stretch these muscles correctly you gain range of motion. This should be felt in the back leg NOT the front leg.

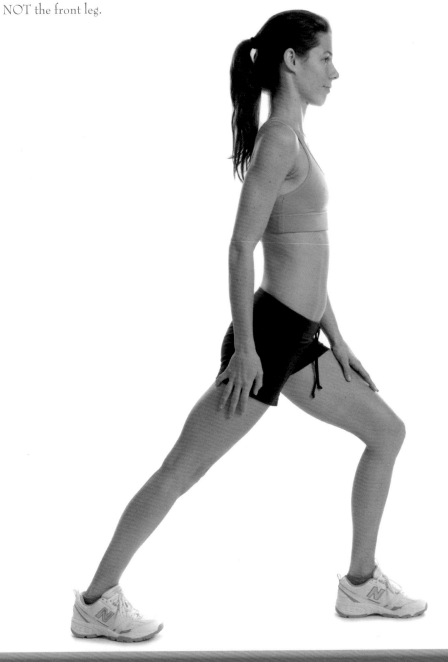

HOW TO DO IT

1 Stand with your legs straight, one foot behind the other.

2 Bring your front leg forward and bend your front knee.

3 Keeping both heels on the floor, lean into your front leg until you feel the stretch in your back calf muscle. Hold for 15 seconds. Repeat sequence three times on each leg.

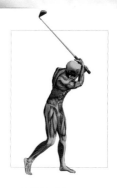

PRIMARY TARGETS
• gastrocnemius

BENEFITS
• Calves

CAUTIONS
• Avoid bending your extended leg.
• Lifting your heel off the floor.

PERFECT YOUR FORM
• Keep your chest upright and lifted as you lean into the stretch

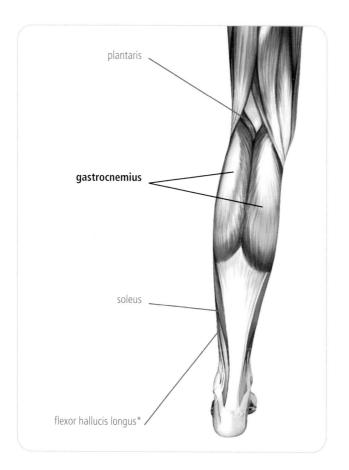

plantaris

gastrocnemius

soleus

flexor hallucis longus*

ANNOTATION KEY

Black text indicates strengthening muscles
Gray text indicates stretching muscles
Italic text indicates tendons and ligaments
- - - - *indicates deep muscles

SOLEUS STRETCH

STRETCH

THE SOLEUS MUSCLES attach to the leg above the ankle, and when you stretch these muscles correctly you gain range of motion. In general, stretches that bend the knee focus on the soleus muscle, while stretches that straighten the knee focus on the gastrocnemius muscle.

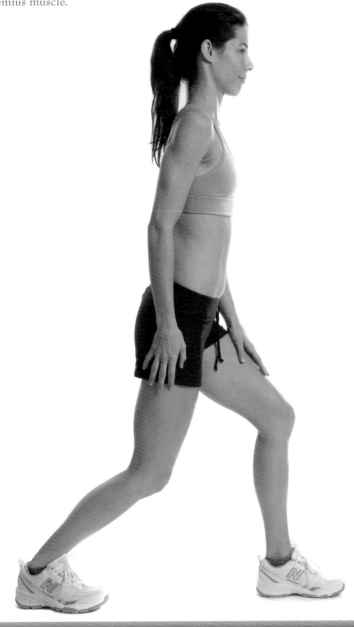

HOW TO DO IT

1 Stand with one foot about one stride length back, knee bent.

2 Bring the other foot forward and bend at the knee.

3 Keeping both heels on the floor, lean into the stretch as you bend your back knee. Once you feel the stretch, hold the position for 15 seconds. Repeat stretch three times. Switch legs and repeat sequence three times.

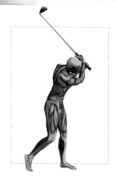

ANNOTATION KEY

Black text indicates strengthening muscles
Gray text indicates stretching muscles
Italic text indicates tendons and ligaments
- - - - *indicates deep muscles

PRIMARY TARGETS
• soleus

BENEFITS
• Calves

CAUTIONS
• Avoid lifting your heel off the floor.

PERFECT YOUR FORM
• Keep your chest upright and lifted as you lean into the stretch.

gastrocnemius

soleus

peroneus

flexor hallucis longus*

GOBLET SQUAT

BEGINNER

THE GOBLET SQUAT targets the quadriceps, calves, glutes and hamstrings. It is especially good for building strength in the quadriceps. Taking a wider stance will reduce the range of motion and make the exercise less demanding, while a closer stance will increase the range and make it more difficult.

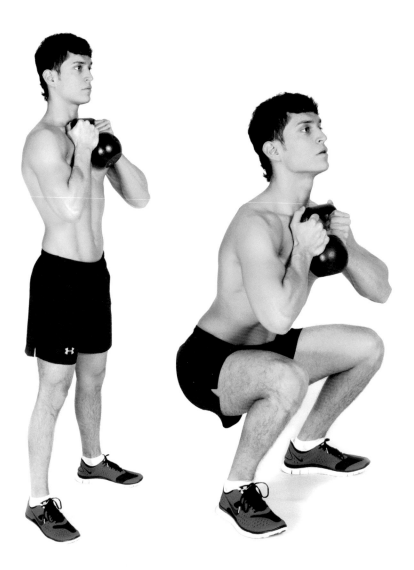

HOW TO DO IT

1 While in a standing position, hold a kettlebell with both hands close to your chest. Your legs should be a little more than shoulder-width apart, with your toes pointing slightly outward.

2 Squat down until your thighs are parallel to the floor, bringing your elbows to your thighs.

3 Keep your back flat as you push through your heels back to the standing position. Complete 8–10 repetitions.

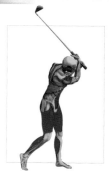

PRIMARY TARGETS
- vastus intermedius
- vastus lateralis
- vastus medialis
- rectus femoris

BENEFITS
- Quadriceps
- Calves
- Glutes
- Hamstrings
- Shoulders

CAUTIONS
- Avoid hyperextending your knees past your toes.

PERFECT YOUR FORM
- Always employ a full range of motion.

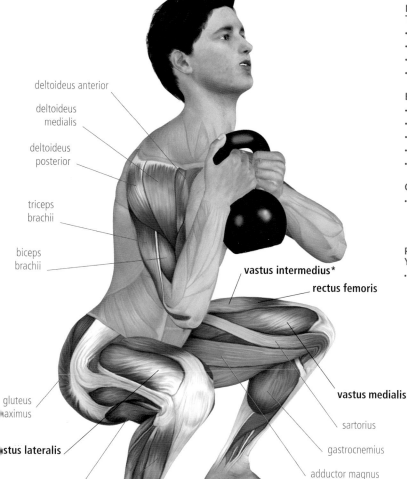

deltoideus anterior

deltoideus medialis

deltoideus posterior

triceps brachii

biceps brachii

vastus intermedius*

rectus femoris

vastus medialis

sartorius

gluteus maximus

gastrocnemius

vastus lateralis

adductor magnus

biceps femoris

tibialis anterior

ANNOTATION KEY

Black text indicates strengthening muscles
Gray text indicates stretching muscles
Italic text indicates tendons and ligaments
- - - - *indicates deep muscles

DEPTH JUMPS

INTERMEDIATE

DEPTH JUMPS BENEFIT the quadriceps, hamstrings, glutes and calves. They improve your speed, power and general athleticism. As a variation, you can use your arms to increase speed or even make the routine more challenging by using higher platforms.

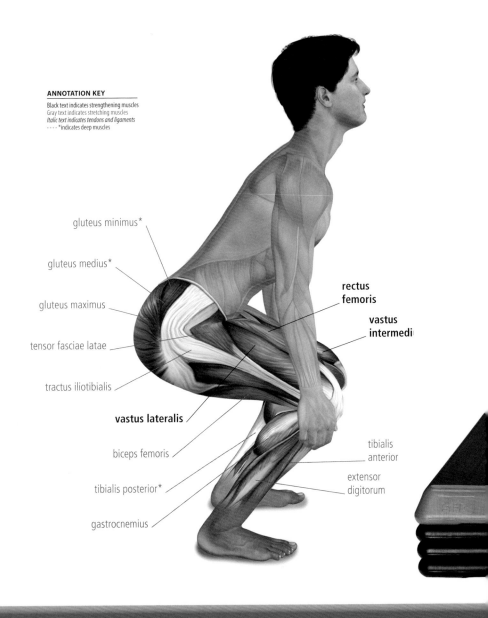

ANNOTATION KEY

Black text indicates strengthening muscles
Gray text indicates stretching muscles
Italic text indicates tendons and ligaments
- - - - *indicates deep muscles

gluteus minimus*

gluteus medius*

gluteus maximus

tensor fasciae latae

tractus iliotibialis

vastus lateralis

biceps femoris

tibialis posterior*

gastrocnemius

rectus femoris

vastus intermedi

tibialis anterior

extensor digitorum

HOW TO DO IT

1 Face two plyo boxes or platforms placed about a metre apart from each other, then stand on top of the one closest to you.

2 Jump off the plyo box; be sure to land between the two boxes on the balls of your feet.

3 As soon as your feet hit the ground, spring up onto the other box.

4 As soon as you land on the second box, turn around and start again. Repeat 15 times.

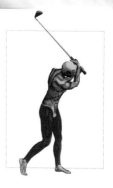

PRIMARY TARGETS
• vastus intermedius
• vastus lateralis
• vastus medialis
• rectus femoris

BENEFITS
• Quadriceps
• Hamstrings
• Glutes
• Calves

CAUTIONS
• Avoid landing on your toes or heels.

PERFECT YOUR FORM
• Be sure to maintain an erect posture throughout the movement.

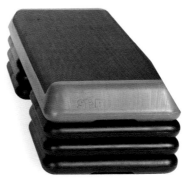

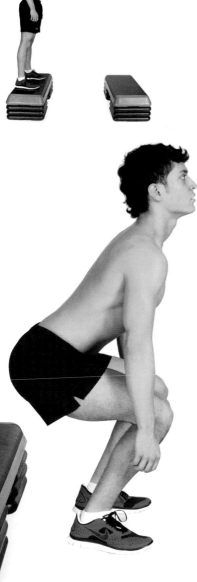

BURPEES

INTERMEDIATE

BURPEES ARE AIMED at the glutes, quadriceps, hamstrings and calves. They serve to increase both muscular strength and endurance. You can make it easier by jumping at a very low height, while adding a push-up to the routine will add an extra level of difficulty.

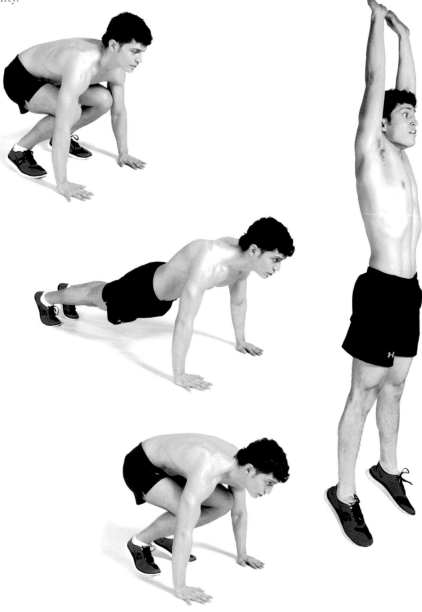

HOW TO DO IT

1 Start in a squat position, with your hands firmly planted on the floor, shoulder-width apart.

2 Kick your feet back and straighten your legs into a push-up position.

3 Quickly return to the squat position.

4 Leap vertically from the squat position as high as possible, raising your arms as you jump. Complete 15 repetitions.

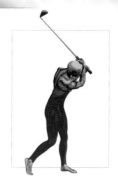

PRIMARY TARGETS
- gluteus maximus
- gluteus minimus
- gluteus medius
- vastus intermedius
- vastus lateralis
- vastus medialis
- rectus femoris

BENEFITS
- Glutes
- Quadriceps
- Hamstrings
- Erectors
- Calves

CAUTIONS
- Avoid landing excessively hard.

PERFECT YOUR FORM
- Be sure to keep a tight core throughout the movement.

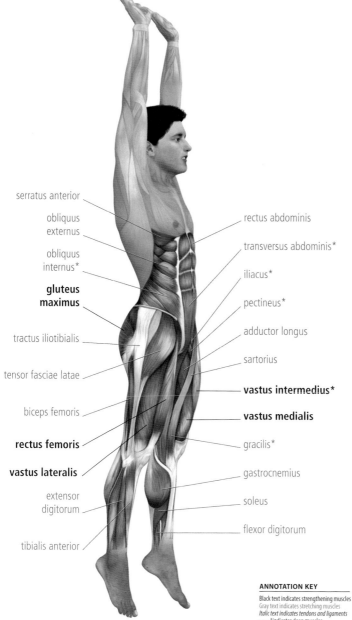

serratus anterior

obliquus externus

obliquus internus*

gluteus maximus

tractus iliotibialis

tensor fasciae latae

biceps femoris

rectus femoris

vastus lateralis

extensor digitorum

tibialis anterior

rectus abdominis

transversus abdominis*

iliacus*

pectineus*

adductor longus

sartorius

vastus intermedius*

vastus medialis

gracilis*

gastrocnemius

soleus

flexor digitorum

ANNOTATION KEY

Black text indicates strengthening muscles
Gray text indicates stretching muscles
Italic text indicates tendons and ligaments
- - - - *indicates deep muscles

CROSSOVER STEPUP

ADVANCED

THIS EXERCISE WORKS the glutes, quads and hamstrings through all planes of motion with a focus on lateral movement. This lateral movement engages the hips in a different way than traditional stepups, involving both internal and external rotation while working on your coordination and balance. Starting with a lower platform may also help you perfect your form.

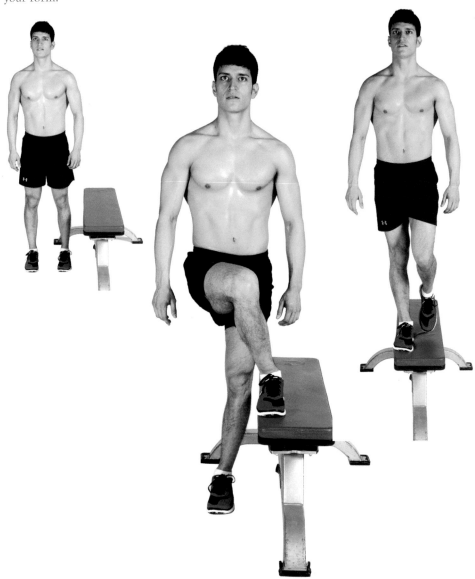

HOW TO DO IT

1 Stand to the right of a bench.

2 Cross your right leg in front of your left and step on to the bench. Push through the stabilised right heel on the bench to raise yourself up.

3 Bring the left leg up onto the bench, then perform the motion in reverse to step down. Repeat 15 times per leg before switching to the other side.

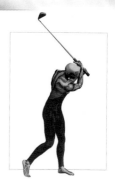

PRIMARY TARGETS
• vastus intermedius
• vastus lateralis
• vastus medialis
• rectus femoris
• semitendinosus
• biceps femoris
• semimembranosus
• gluteus maximus
• gluteus minimus
• gluteus medius

BENEFITS
• Quadriceps
• Hamstrings
• Glutes
• Core

CAUTIONS
• Avoid hyperextending your knee past your toes.

PERFECT YOUR FORM
• Maintain an erect posture throughout the movement.

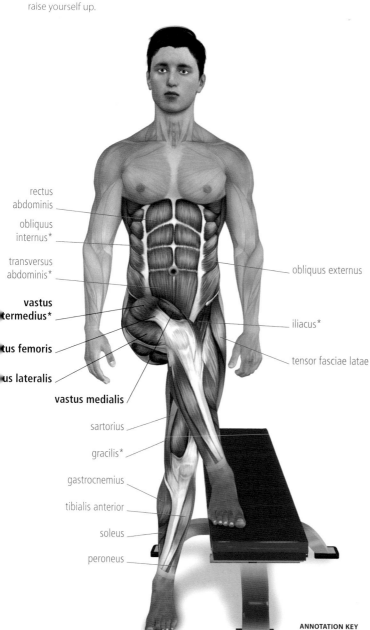

rectus abdominis

obliquus internus*

transversus abdominis*

vastus intermedius*

rectus femoris

vastus lateralis

vastus medialis

sartorius

gracilis*

gastrocnemius

tibialis anterior

soleus

peroneus

obliquus externus

iliacus*

tensor fasciae latae

ANNOTATION KEY

Black text indicates strengthening muscles
Gray text indicates stretching muscles
Italic text indicates tendons and ligaments
---- *indicates deep muscles

CHAIR SQUAT

INTERMEDIATE

The Chair Squat is a lunge variation with a shortened range of motion. It is a strength builder for the legs but also develops the balance required for many sports. Slow movement in the motion plays a critical factor in its proper execution.

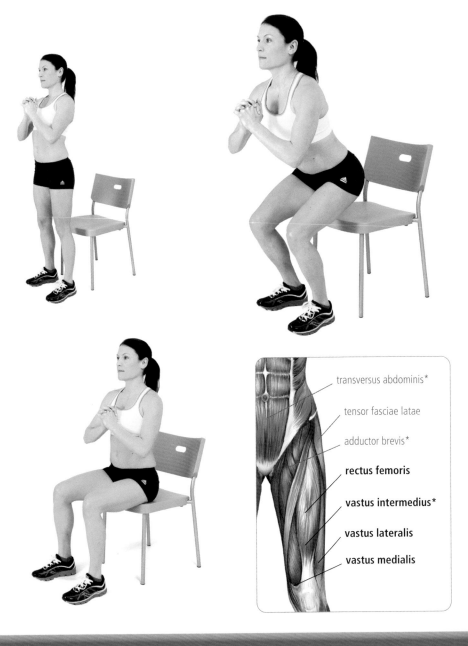

transversus abdominis*

tensor fasciae latae

adductor brevis*

rectus femoris

vastus intermedius*

vastus lateralis

vastus medialis

HOW TO DO IT

1 Stand upright in front of the chair. Clasp your hands and position them in front of your chest.

2 Slowly lower into a squat position.

3 Continue lowering until you are resting on the chair.

4 With control, rise back up to the starting position and repeat, aiming for 10 repetitions.

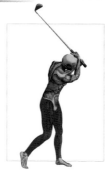

ANNOTATION KEY

Black text indicates strengthening muscles
Gray text indicates stretching muscles
Italic text indicates tendons and ligaments
- - - - *indicates deep muscles

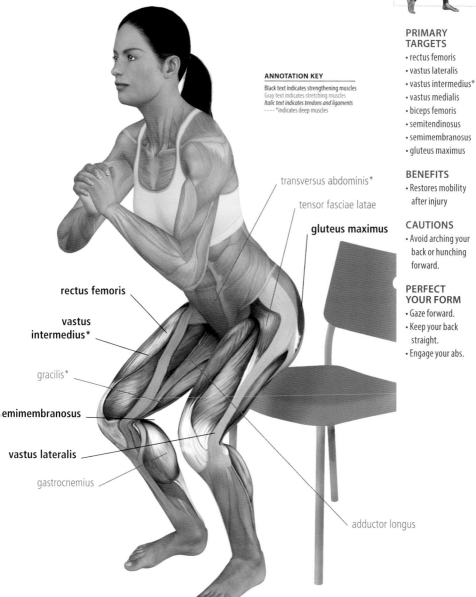

transversus abdominis*

tensor fasciae latae

gluteus maximus

rectus femoris

vastus intermedius*

gracilis*

emimembranosus

vastus lateralis

gastrocnemius

adductor longus

PRIMARY TARGETS

- rectus femoris
- vastus lateralis
- vastus intermedius*
- vastus medialis
- biceps femoris
- semitendinosus
- semimembranosus
- gluteus maximus

BENEFITS

- Restores mobility after injury

CAUTIONS

- Avoid arching your back or hunching forward.

PERFECT YOUR FORM

- Gaze forward.
- Keep your back straight.
- Engage your abs.

MOUNTAIN CLIMBER

BEGINNER

THE MOUNTAIN CLIMBER is a stability exercise that also tests and extends the endurance and the activation of many muscles working together to execute the movement. This is a taxing and repetitious exercise that, quite simply, works.

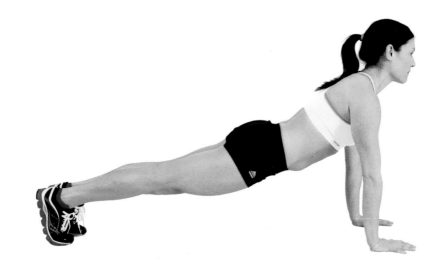

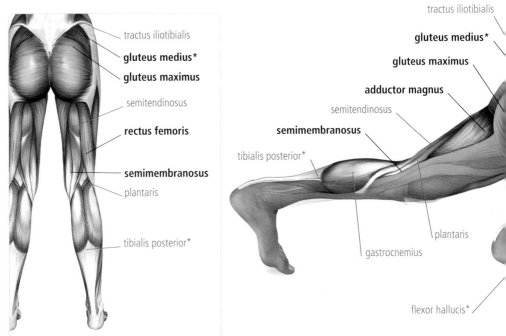

tractus iliotibialis

gluteus medius*

gluteus maximus

semitendinosus

rectus femoris

semimembranosus

plantaris

tibialis posterior*

tractus iliotibialis

gluteus medius*

gluteus maximus

adductor magnus

semitendinosus

semimembranosus

tibialis posterior*

plantaris

gastrocnemius

flexor hallucis*

HOW TO DO IT

1 Begin in an upper pushup position, palms and toes on the floor.

2 Bring your right knee in toward your chest. Rest the ball of the foot on the floor.

3 Jump to switch feet in the air, bringing the left foot in and the right foot back. Continue alternating your feet as fast as you can safely go for 30 to 60 seconds.

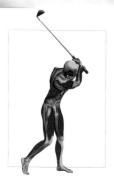

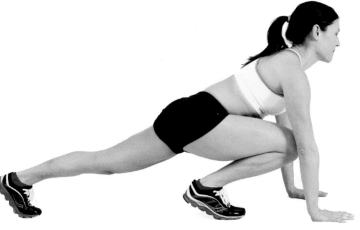

PRIMARY TARGETS
• vastus lateralis
• rectus femoris
• gluteus maximus
• gluteus medius*
• semimembranosus
• adductor magnus
• levator scapulae*
• splenius*
• trapezius

BENEFITS
• Strengthens and tones abdominal, chest, and leg muscles

CAUTIONS
• Avoid moving through the positions so quickly that you compromise your form.

PERFECT YOUR FORM
• As much as possible, keep your hands planted on the floor.

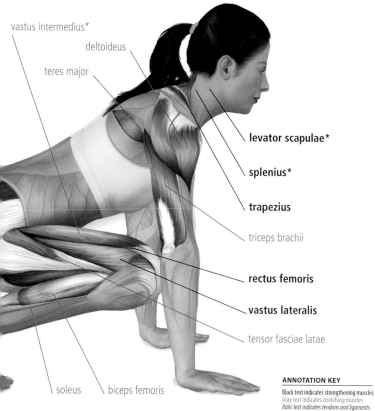

vastus intermedius*

deltoideus

teres major

levator scapulae*

splenius*

trapezius

triceps brachii

rectus femoris

vastus lateralis

tensor fasciae latae

soleus

biceps femoris

ANNOTATION KEY

Black text indicates strengthening muscles
Gray text indicates stretching muscles
Italic text indicates tendons and ligaments
---- *indicates deep muscles

SWISS BALL BRIDGING RAISE

ADVANCED

THE SWISS BALL Bridging Raise targets the hamstrings, glutes and abs. It increases power in the hamstrings, particularly the semitendinosus, biceps femoris and semimembranosus muscles.

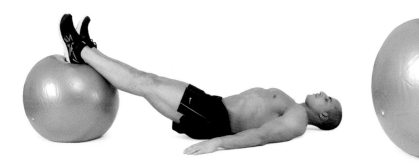

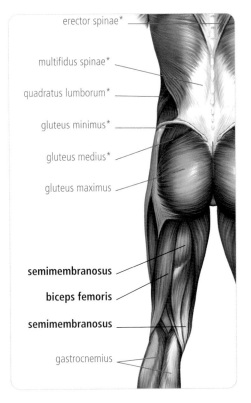

erector spinae*

multifidus spinae*

quadratus lumborum*

gluteus minimus*

gluteus medius*

gluteus maximus

semimembranosus

biceps femoris

semimembranosus

gastrocnemius

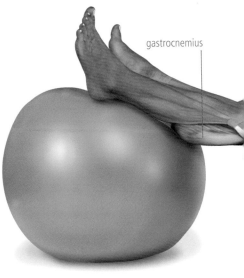

gastrocnemius

HOW TO DO IT

1 Lie face-up on the floor with your arms at your sides and your lower legs resting on the Swiss ball.

2 Press your palms into the floor and engage your abdominal muscles as you lift your upper body off the floor. Your body should form a diagonal line. If desired, hold for a few seconds.

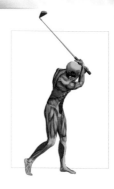

PRIMARY TARGETS

- extensor carpi radialis
- extensor carpi ulnaris
- extensor digiti minimi
- extensor digitorum
- extensor indicis
- extensor pollicis

BENEFITS

- Wrists
- Hands
- Forearms

CAUTIONS

- Avoid lifting or tensing your shoulders.

PERFECT YOUR FORM

- Be sure to press your thumb into the meaty part of your palm, attached to the thumb, intensifying the stretch in your forearm and wrist.

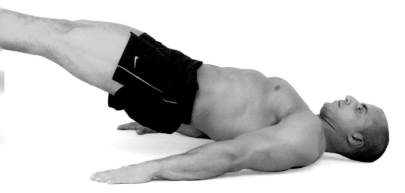

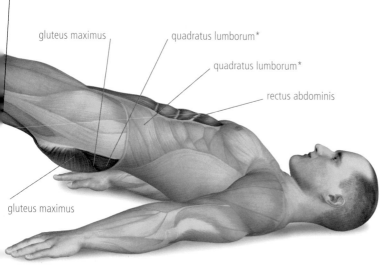

rectus femoris

gluteus maximus

quadratus lumborum*

quadratus lumborum*

rectus abdominis

gluteus maximus

ANNOTATION KEY

Black text indicates strengthening muscles
Gray text indicates stretching muscles
Italic text indicates tendons and ligaments
- - - - *indicates deep muscles

LATERAL LOW LUNGE

BEGINNER

The Lateral Low Lunge concentrates on the gluteal and thigh muscles. It is excellent for strengthening the pelvic, trunk, and knee stabilizers. It is not advisable if you have sharp knee pain, back pain or trouble bearing weight on one leg.

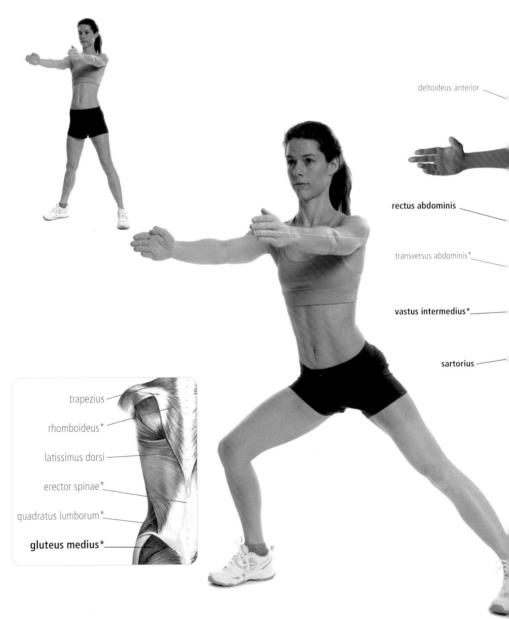

deltoideus anterior

rectus abdominis

transversus abdominis*

vastus intermedius*

sartorius

trapezius

rhomboideus*

latissimus dorsi

erector spinae*

quadratus lumborum*

gluteus medius*

HOW TO DO IT

1 Stand with your feet planted widely and your arms outstretched in front of you, parallel to the floor.

2 Step out to the left. Squat down on your right leg, bending at your hips, while maintaining a neutral spine. Begin to extend your left leg, keeping both feet flat on the floor.

3 Bend your right knee until your thigh is parallel to the floor, and your left leg is fully extended.

4 Keeping your arms parallel to the ground, squeeze your buttocks and press off your right leg to return to the starting position, and repeat. Repeat sequence 10 times on each side.

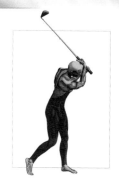

PRIMARY TARGETS
- adductor longus
- adductor magnus
- semitendinosus
- semimembranosus
- biceps femoris
- sartorius
- vastus medialis
- vastus lateralis
- vastus intermedius
- rectus femoris
- gluteus maximus
- gluteus medius
- rectus abdominis

BENEFITS
- Gluteal area
- Quadriceps

CAUTIONS
- Avoid craning your neck as you perform the movement.
- Lifting your feet off the floor.

PERFECT YOUR FORM
- Keep your spine in neutral position as you bend your hips.
- Relax your shoulders and neck.

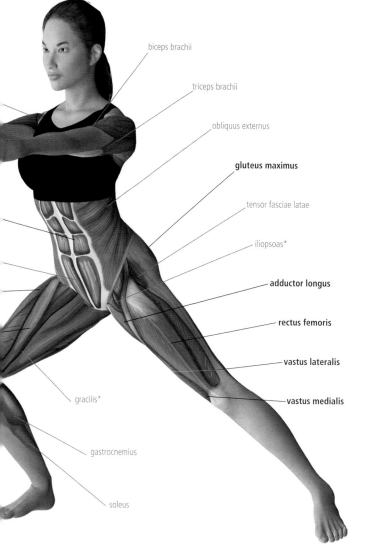

biceps brachii

triceps brachii

obliquus externus

gluteus maximus

tensor fasciae latae

iliopsoas*

adductor longus

rectus femoris

vastus lateralis

vastus medialis

gracilis*

gastrocnemius

soleus

ANNOTATION KEY

Black text indicates strengthening muscles
Gray text indicates stretching muscles
Italic text indicates tendons and ligaments
- - - - *indicates deep muscles

HIP EXTENSION AND FLEXION

BEGINNER

THESE EXERCISES ARE an advanced version of the classic leg extension, which places emphasis on the core as well as the legs. An effective leg-strengthener as well as a stabilizer, this is particularly effective for isolating the individual sections of the leg muscles.

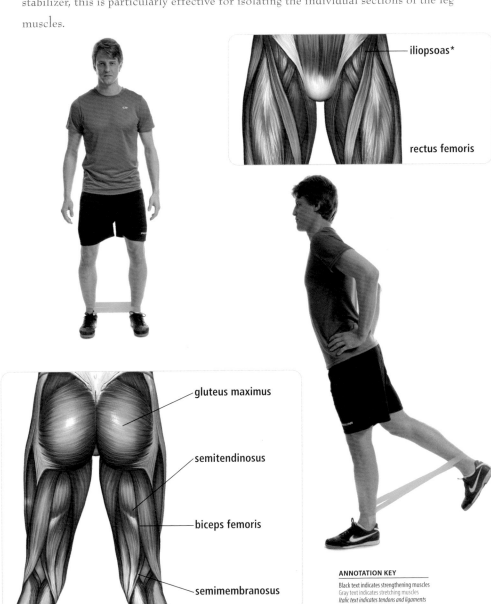

iliopsoas*

rectus femoris

gluteus maximus

semitendinosus

biceps femoris

semimembranosus

ANNOTATION KEY

Black text indicates strengthening muscles
Gray text indicates stretching muscles
Italic text indicates tendons and ligaments
- - - - *indicates deep muscles

HOW TO DO IT

1 Stand with your feet shoulder-width apart, with a resistance loop or a resistance band tied around your ankles. Tuck your pelvis slightly forward, lift your chest and press your shoulders downward and back.

2 Keeping your head up, shoulders back and hands on your hips, slowly extend your leg backwards.

3 Perform three sets of 10 repetitions, and return to the starting position.

4 Switch legs, and repeat on the other side.

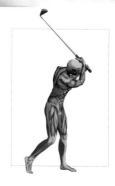

PRIMARY TARGETS
• rectus femoris
• iliopsoas
• gluteus maximus
• biceps femoris
• semitendinosus
• semimembranosus

BENEFITS
• Hip extensors
• Hip flexors

CAUTIONS
• Avoid bending your knee.
• Allowing your hips to shift out of line.

PERFECT YOUR FORM
• Tighten your glutes as you move your leg backward during the extension phase of the exercise.
• Tighten the muscles at the front of your thigh and hip as you move your leg forward during the flexion phase of the exercise.

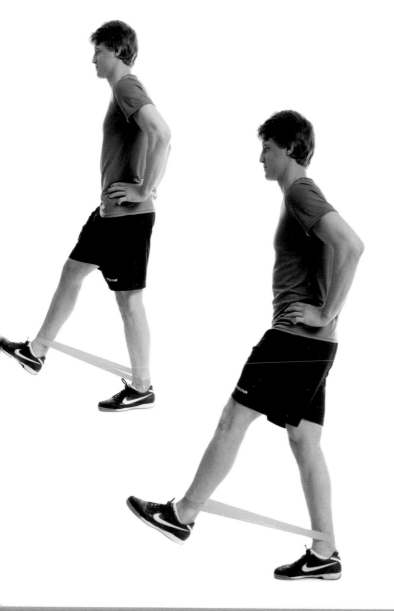

LATERAL EXTENSION REVERSE LUNGE

INTERMEDIATE

THIS EXERCISE IS one of the most effective leg-strengthening exercises. Working through an explosive full range of motion, the Lateral Extension Reverse Lunge is to the legs what the Barbell Curl is to the arms.

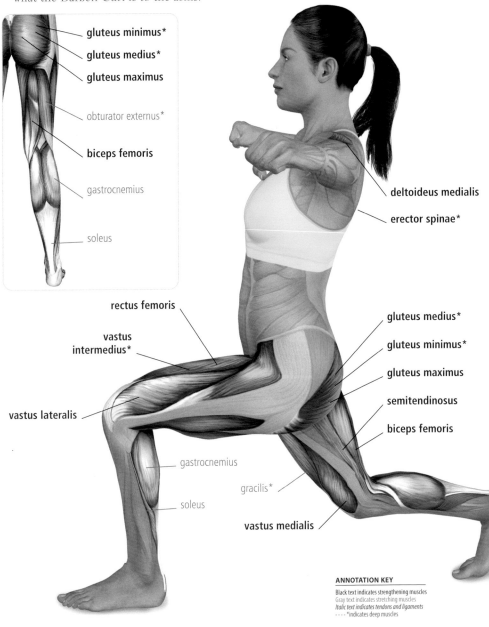

gluteus minimus*

gluteus medius*

gluteus maximus

obturator externus*

biceps femoris

gastrocnemius

soleus

deltoideus medialis

erector spinae*

rectus femoris

vastus intermedius*

vastus lateralis

gastrocnemius

gracilis*

soleus

vastus medialis

gluteus medius*

gluteus minimus*

gluteus maximus

semitendinosus

biceps femoris

ANNOTATION KEY

Black text indicates strengthening muscles
Gray text indicates stretching muscles
Italic text indicates tendons and ligaments
---- *indicates deep muscles

HOW TO DO IT

1 Stand with your feet hip-width apart and your arms at your sides or on your hips.

2 Step your right leg back, resting the bottom of the foot on the floor.

3 Bend both knees as you move into a lunge position. Lower your body, flexing your left knee and hip until your right leg is almost in contact with the floor. Raise your arms to the side until they are level with your shoulders.

4 Return to starting position by extending the hip and knee of your left leg and bringing your right leg forward to meet your left.

5 Repeat on the opposite side. Alternating, complete 10 on each side.

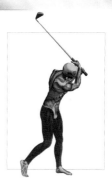

PRIMARY TARGETS

- rectus femoris
- vastus lateralis
- vastus intermedius*
- vastus medialis
- biceps femoris
- semitendinosus
- semimembranosus
- gluteus maximus
- gluteus medius*
- gluteus minimus*
- deltoideus medialis
- erector spinae*

BENEFITS

- Strengthens gluteal and leg muscles

CAUTIONS

- Avoid twisting either hip.
- Hunching your shoulders.
- Arching your back or hunching forward.

PERFECT YOUR FORM

- Keep your shoulders pressed downward.

CHAIR PLIÉ

INTERMEDIATE

THE CHAIR PLIÉ is beneficial for the quadriceps, hamstrings, glutes and core. It serves to increase power and mass in the thighs. To increase the difficulty level, place your feet farther apart as this increases the effort required to complete the squat.

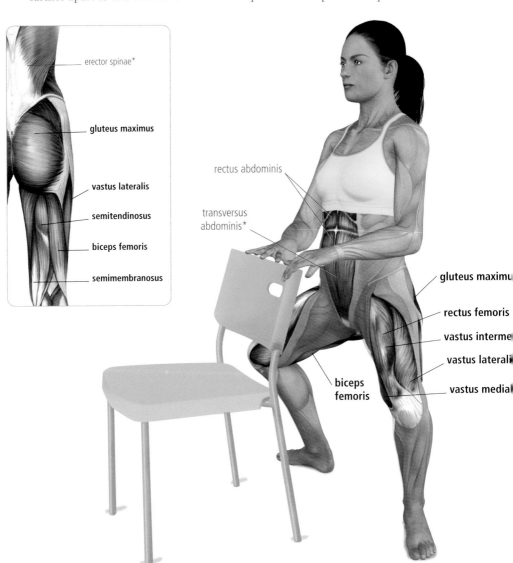

erector spinae*

gluteus maximus

vastus lateralis

semitendinosus

biceps femoris

semimembranosus

rectus abdominis

transversus
abdominis*

gluteus maximu

rectus femoris

vastus interme

vastus laterali

biceps
femoris

vastus media

ANNOTATION KEY

Black text indicates strengthening muscles
Gray text indicates stretching muscles
Italic text indicates tendons and ligaments
- - - - *indicates deep muscles

HOW TO DO IT

1 Stand with your feet in a wide stance, with toes turned out and the chair in front of you.

2 Keeping your knees aligned with your toes, bend your knees and lower your body into a squat position.

3 Keeping your back straight, raise yourself back to starting position. Perform 10 repetitions.

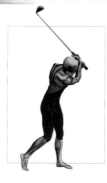

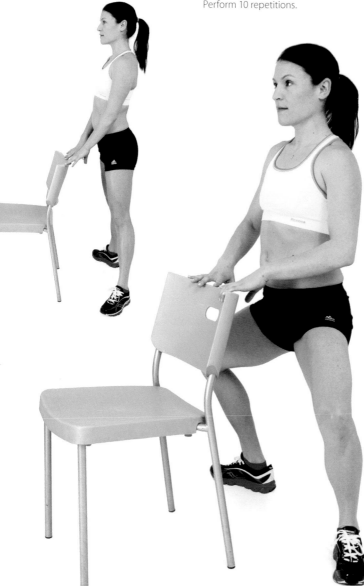

PRIMARY TARGETS
• gluteus maximus
• rectus femoris
• vastus lateralis
• vastus intermedius*
• vastus medialis
• biceps femoris
• semitendinosus
• semimembranosus

BENEFITS
• Engages and tones inner-thigh adductors

CAUTIONS
• Avoid turning your toes out to the point where it is uncomfortable.

PERFECT YOUR FORM
• Keep your abdominal muscles pulled in.

BARBELL SQUAT

INTERMEDIATE

THE ICONIC BARBELL SQUAT is one of the most effective strengthening exercises you can take on. It is fantastic for strengthening the lower body and the core and has a positive effect on your metabolism.

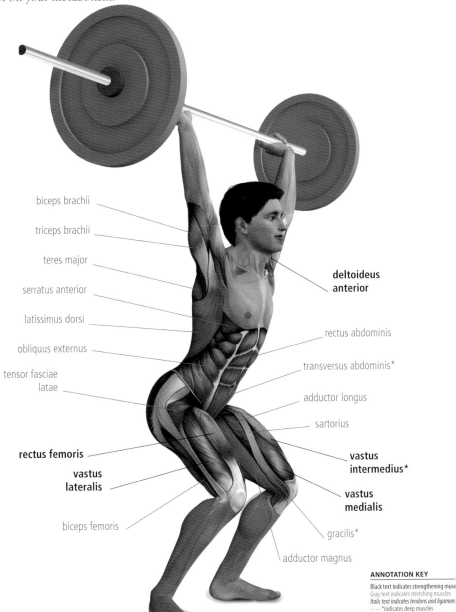

biceps brachii

triceps brachii

teres major

serratus anterior

latissimus dorsi

obliquus externus

tensor fasciae latae

rectus femoris

vastus lateralis

biceps femoris

deltoideus anterior

rectus abdominis

transversus abdominis*

adductor longus

sartorius

vastus intermedius*

vastus medialis

gracilis*

adductor magnus

ANNOTATION KEY

Black text indicates strengthening musc⟨
Gray text indicates stretching muscles
*Italic text indicates tendons and ligamen⟩
- - - - *indicates deep muscles

HOW TO DO IT

1 Begin standing with your feet shoulder-width apart in front of a barbell. Squat down and grab the barbell with a wide overhand grip. Make sure your knees are close to the bar.

2 As you return to a standing position, flip the barbell directly overhead with your arms locked.

3 Stand fully erect while holding the completed movement overhead.

4 Lower the barbell carefully to your chest and then down to the ground. Perform 6–8 repetitions.

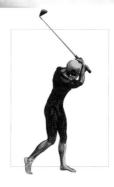

PRIMARY TARGETS

- deltoideus anterior
- deltoideus medialis
- deltoideus posterior
- vastus intermedius
- vastus lateralis
- vastus medialis
- rectus femoris
- gluteus maximus
- gluteus medius
- gluteus minimus

BENEFITS

- Deltoids
- Thighs
- Glutes
- Upper back
- Core
- Triceps
- Hamstrings

CAUTIONS

- Avoid overarching your back.

PERFECT YOUR FORM

- Increases power and mass in the shoulders and thighs.

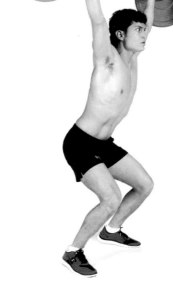
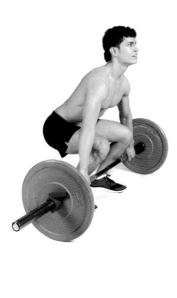
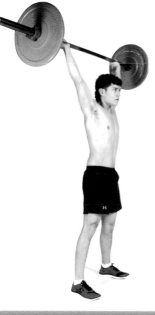
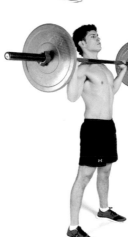

SPLIT SQUAT WITH OVERHEAD PRESS

ADVANCED

THE SPLIT SQUAT IS an easy way of strengthening the glutes and thighs. It also improves balance; helps to stabilize the pelvis, trunk and knees; and boosts general movement strength.

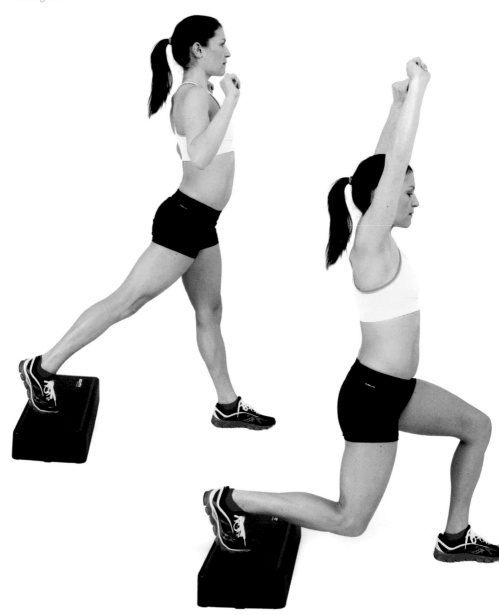

HOW TO DO IT

1 Stand with your right leg behind you, with the ball of the foot resting on a step.

2 With your elbows bent to form right angles, raise both arms to shoulder height.

3 Bend both knees into a split squat position. Simultaneously, extend your arms over your head.

4 Return to starting position, and then repeat. Aim for 10 repetitions. Then, switch sides and perform 10 more repetitions with the other leg behind. If desired, repeat the whole sequence 2 more times.

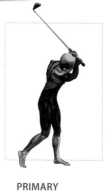

PRIMARY TARGETS

- rectus femoris
- vastus lateralis
- vastus intermedius*
- vastus medialis
- biceps femoris
- semitendinosus
- semimembranosus
- gluteus maximus
- gluteus medius*
- gluteus minimus*
- deltoideus anterior
- deltoideus medialis
- deltoideus posterior

BENEFITS

- Strengthens glutes, quadriceps, hamstrings and trapezius

CAUTIONS

- Avoid arching your back as you raise your arms.

PERFECT YOUR FORM

- Keep your back straight and your core upright.

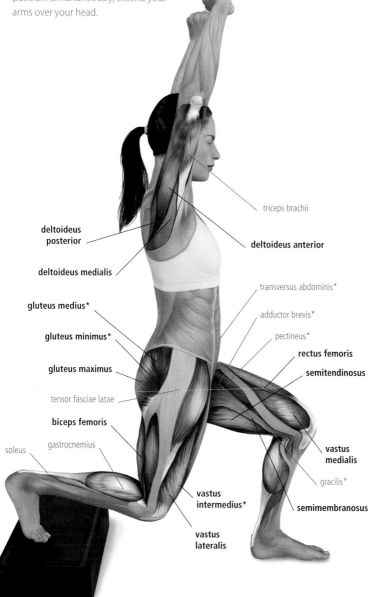

triceps brachii

deltoideus anterior

transversus abdominis*

adductor brevis*

pectineus*

rectus femoris

semitendinosus

vastus medialis

gracilis*

semimembranosus

deltoideus posterior

deltoideus medialis

gluteus medius*

gluteus minimus*

gluteus maximus

tensor fasciae latae

biceps femoris

gastrocnemius

soleus

vastus intermedius*

vastus lateralis

JUMPING LUNGE

ADVANCED

THE JUMPING LUNGE is a great strengthening exercise for your quadriceps and also your glutes and calves. By keeping the tension on the intended muscles throughout the movement, this exercise will effectively work the quadriceps through a full range of motion.

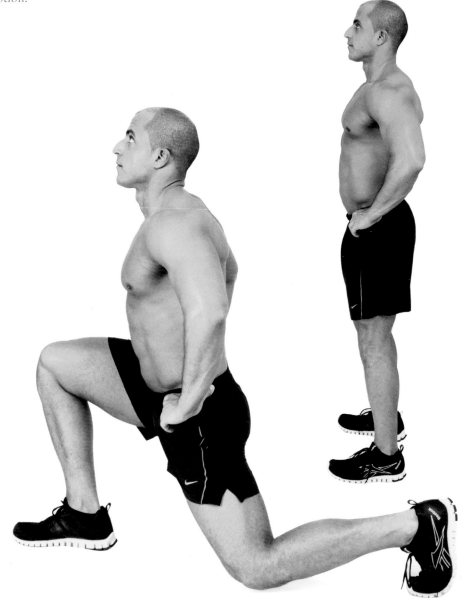

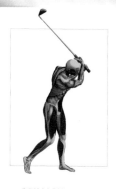

HOW TO DO IT

1 Stand upright, with your feet hip-width apart and your hands on your hips.

2 With your right leg, take a big step forward.

3 Bend both legs to lower into a deep lunge. Then, straighten both legs.

4 Jump up to switch legs so that your left leg is in front. Take a moment to find your balance.

5 Bend both knees to sink down into another lunge. Straighten your knees and then repeat, performing 10 repetitions.

PRIMARY TARGETS

- rectus femoris
- vastus lateralis
- vastus intermedius*
- vastus medialis
- biceps femoris
- semitendinosus
- semimembranosus
- gastrocnemius
- gluteus maximus
- gluteus medius*
- gluteus minimus*

BENEFITS

- Plyometrically integrates explosive movement with coordinated agility training

CAUTIONS

- Avoid allowing your front knee to twist to either side.

PERFECT YOUR FORM

- Keep breathing throughout the exercise.

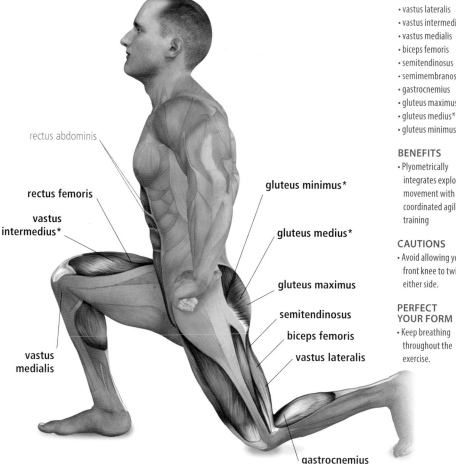

rectus abdominis

rectus femoris

vastus intermedius*

vastus medialis

gluteus minimus*

gluteus medius*

gluteus maximus

semitendinosus

biceps femoris

vastus lateralis

gastrocnemius

ANNOTATION KEY

Black text indicates strengthening muscles
Gray text indicates stretching muscles
Italic text indicates tendons and ligaments
---- *indicates deep muscles

ONE-LEGGED STEP DOWN

INTERMEDIATE

THIS HIPS, BUTT AND THIGH exercise is perfect for targeting the major muscles of the lower body but may require some practice to get your form down. The exercise can be modified by holding a dumbbell or kettlebell in each hand.

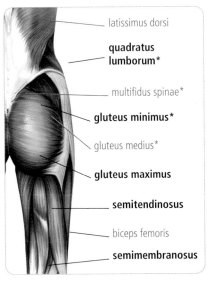

- latissimus dorsi
- **quadratus lumborum***
- multifidus spinae*
- **gluteus minimus***
- gluteus medius*
- **gluteus maximus**
- **semitendinosus**
- biceps femoris
- **semimembranosus**

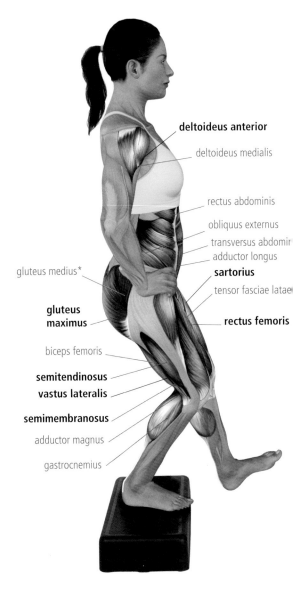

- **deltoideus anterior**
- deltoideus medialis
- rectus abdominis
- obliquus externus
- transversus abdomin
- adductor longus
- **sartorius**
- tensor fasciae latae
- **rectus femoris**
- gluteus medius*
- **gluteus maximus**
- biceps femoris
- **semitendinosus**
- **vastus lateralis**
- **semimembranosus**
- adductor magnus
- gastrocnemius

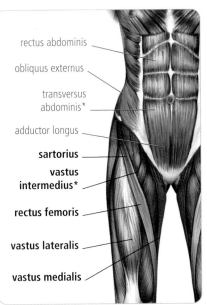

- rectus abdominis
- obliquus externus
- transversus abdominis*
- adductor longus
- **sartorius**
- **vastus intermedius***
- **rectus femoris**
- **vastus lateralis**
- **vastus medialis**

HOW TO DO IT

1 Stand facing forward on a step.

2 Bend your right leg. Simultaneously step your left leg downward, flexing the foot to rest on your heel.

3 Without rotating your torso or knee, press upward through your right leg to return to starting position. Switch legs and repeat, performing 20 repetitions.

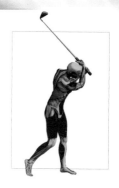

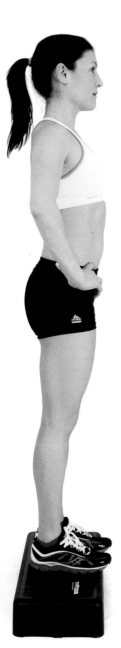

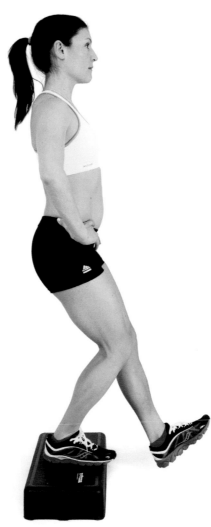

PRIMARY TARGETS
- deltoideus anterior
- quadratus lumborum*
- vastus lateralis
- vastus intermedius*
- vastus medialis
- sartorius
- rectus femoris
- gluteus maximus
- semitendinosus
- semimembranosus

BENEFITS
- Strengthens pelvic and knee stabilisers

CAUTIONS
- Avoid allowing your knee to twist inward; instead, keep it in line with your middle toe.

PERFECT YOUR FORM
- Hold the wall or a rail for support if desired.

ANNOTATION KEY

Black text indicates strengthening muscles
Gray text indicates stretching muscles
Italic text indicates tendons and ligaments
- - - - *indicates deep muscles

REACH-AND-TWIST WALKING LUNGE

ADVANCED

THIS LUNGE CONCENTRATES on the gluteal and thigh muscles. It is excellent for strengthening the pelvic, trunk and knee stabilizers. It is not advisable if you have sharp knee pain, back pain or trouble bearing weight on one leg.

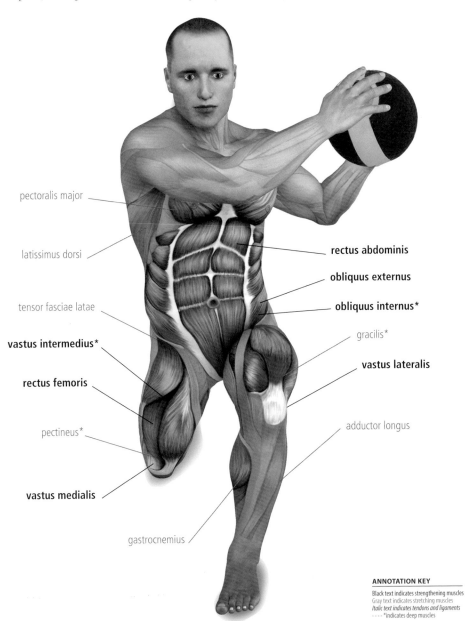

pectoralis major

latissimus dorsi

tensor fasciae latae

vastus intermedius*

rectus femoris

pectineus*

vastus medialis

gastrocnemius

rectus abdominis

obliquus externus

obliquus internus*

gracilis*

vastus lateralis

adductor longus

ANNOTATION KEY

Black text indicates strengthening muscles
Gray text indicates stretching muscles
Italic text indicates tendons and ligaments
- - - - *indicates deep muscles

HOW TO DO IT

1 Stand with feet roughly hip-width apart and your torso facing forward. Hold a weighted medicine ball in both hands.

2 Lunge your left foot forward. Begin to bend both knees, lowering your whole body into the lunge. At the same time, raise the medicine ball until it is over your left shoulder, held in both hands.

3 In a single motion, rise up to stand, bring the ball back to centre, and then perform the lunge and reach in the other direction.

4 Continue to lunge and move the ball from side to side as you walk forward. Continue for 15 steps.

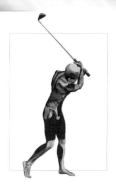

PRIMARY TARGETS

- rectus femoris
- vastus lateralis
- vastus intermedius*
- vastus medialis
- gluteus maximus
- biceps femoris
- semitendinosus
- semimembranosus
- rectus abdominis
- obliquus externus
- obliquus internus*

BENEFITS

- Strengthens and tones core, especially abdominal and gluteal muscles

CAUTIONS

- Avoid hunching your shoulders.
- Arching your back.

PERFECT YOUR FORM

- As much as possible, keep your torso facing forward.

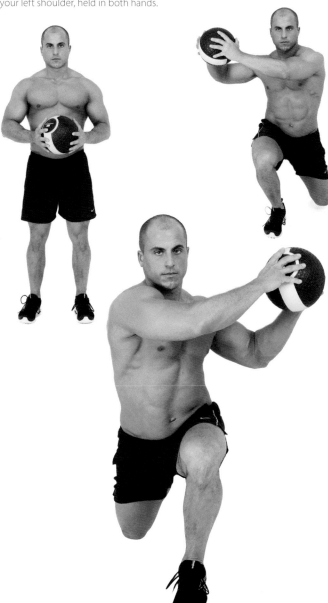

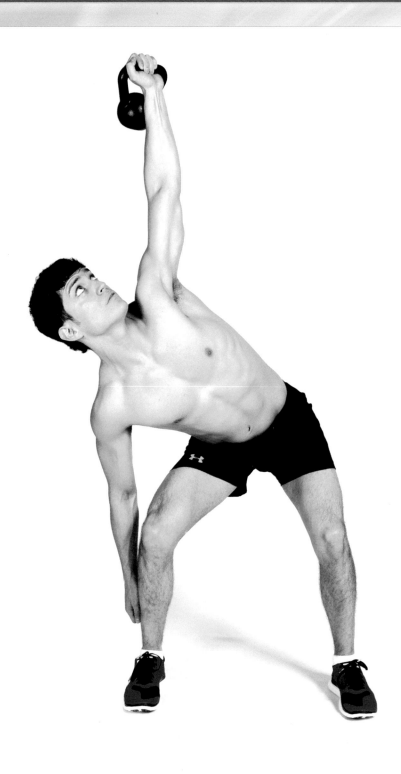

CORE

Your "core" is, very basically, your midsection—all the muscles, bones and ligaments from above the thighs to below the shoulders. Without strong, pliable muscles in your stomach, hips, butt and lower back, you can't make a golf swing that is both powerful and technically sound. Strengthen your core using the exercises in this chapter and you'll notice a dramatic improvement in your golf swing (and potentially more yards through a greater coil).

COBRA STRETCH

STRETCH

THE COBRA is so important in the development of your flexibility. Always start off with the simple back bends, and eventually move toward more difficult poses. Spend time in the Cobra pose, working the muscles of your upper back to open your chest. To check if you are accessing those muscles, try taking some of the weight out of your hands and see if you can still hold the pose.

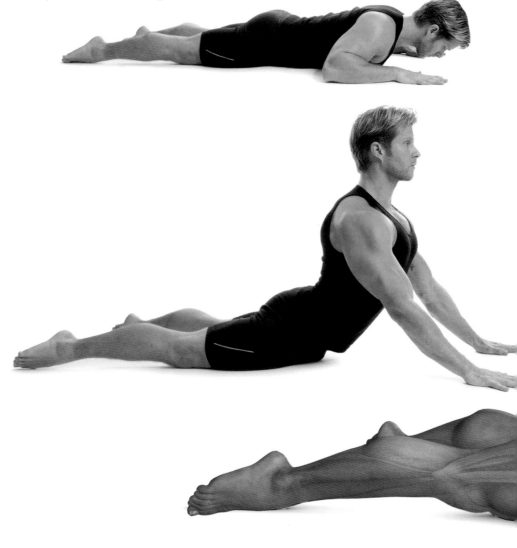

HOW TO DO IT

1 Lie facedown, legs extended behind you with toes pointed. Position the palms of your hands on the floor slightly above your shoulders, and rest your elbows on the floor.

2 Push down into the floor, and slowly lift through the top of your chest as you straighten your arms.

3 Pull your tailbone down toward your pubis as you push your shoulders down and back.

4 Elongate your neck and gaze forward.

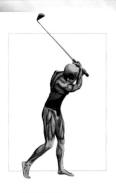

PRIMARY TARGETS
• rectus abdominis
• transversus abdominis
• obliquus externus
• obliquus internus

BENEFITS
• Abdominals

CAUTIONS
• Avoid tipping your head too far backward.
• Overdoing this stretch—it can lead to excessive pressure on your lower back.

PERFECT YOUR FORM
• Maintain pressure between the floor and your hips.
• Relax your shoulders, and keep them down and away from your ears.

ANNOTATION KEY
Black text indicates strengthening muscles
Gray text indicates stretching muscles
Italic text indicates tendons and ligaments
- - - - indicates deep muscles

obliquus externus

rectus abdominis

obliquus internus*

transversus abdominis*

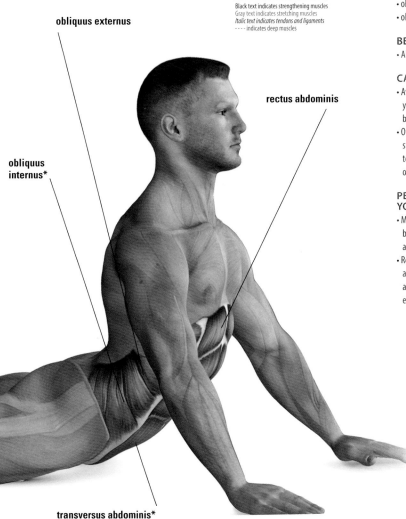

SIDE-LYING RIB STRETCH

INTERMEDIATE

SIDE-STRETCHING EXERCISES lengthen the muscles between the ribs and pelvis—including parts of the lower back—and open the sides of the rib cage, improving rib cage mobility and the expansiveness of the lungs, which makes breathing easier in all situations.

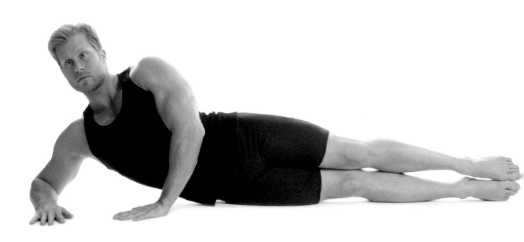

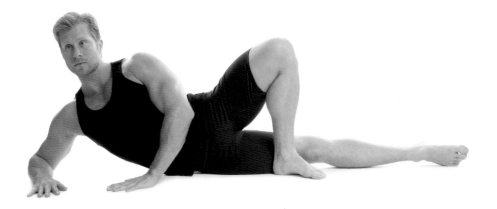

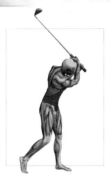

HOW TO DO IT

1 Lie on your right side with your legs together and extended. Place both palms on the floor, your right arm supporting you and your left arm positioned in front of your body. Your upper body should be slightly lifted.

2 Bend your left leg and rest the foot just in front of your right thigh, knee pointing up toward the ceiling.

3 Keeping your legs in place, press down with your hands and straighten both arms as you raise your body upward, feeling a stretch around your right rib cage.

4 Release, switch sides, and repeat.

PRIMARY TARGETS
- obliquus externus
- obliquus internus
- tensor fasciae latae
- multifidus spinae
- erector spinae

BENEFITS
- Rib cage
- Obliques
- Outer thighs
- Lower back

CAUTIONS
- Avoid tightening your jaw, which can cause tension in your neck.

PERFECT YOUR FORM
- Shift your weight forward on your supporting hip.
- Place a towel under your bottom hip if it feels uncomfortable to rest directly on the floor.

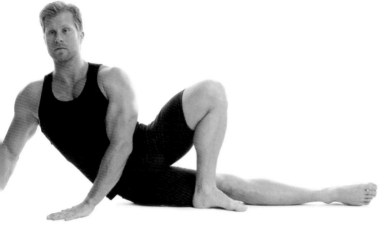

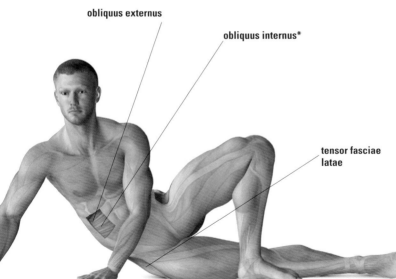

obliquus externus

obliquus internus*

tensor fasciae latae

ANNOTATION KEY
Black text indicates strengthening muscles
Gray text indicates stretching muscles
Italic text indicates tendons and ligaments
- - - - *indicates deep muscles

ADVANCED KETTLEBELL WINDMILL

ADVANCED

THIS IS A VERY TOUGH exercise that is hard to master. Once you have mastered it, you can increase the weight of the kettlebells, and the difficulty returns! It's a total-body strength exercise that especially challenges your shoulders, core, glutes and hamstrings. Try it today—and you're sure to be sore tomorrow.

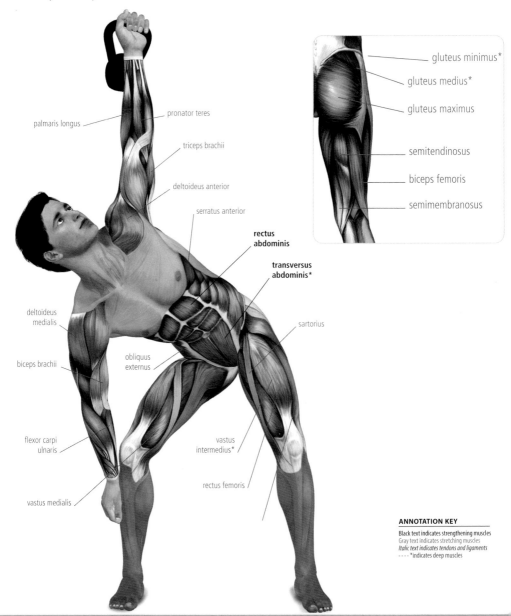

palmaris longus

pronator teres

triceps brachii

deltoideus anterior

serratus anterior

rectus abdominis

transversus abdominis*

deltoideus medialis

biceps brachii

obliquus externus

sartorius

flexor carpi ulnaris

vastus intermedius*

vastus medialis

rectus femoris

gluteus minimus*

gluteus medius*

gluteus maximus

semitendinosus

biceps femoris

semimembranosus

ANNOTATION KEY

Black text indicates strengthening muscles
Gray text indicates stretching muscles
Italic text indicates tendons and ligaments
- - - - *indicates deep muscles

HOW TO DO IT

1 With your right arm by your side and your feet shoulder-width apart, stand with a kettlebell in your left hand, raised overhead.

2 Push your left hip out to the left and slightly bend your knees while lowering your torso to the right as far as possible. Pause, then return to the starting position. Complete 8–10 repetitions per side.

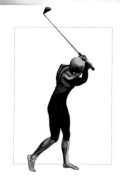

PRIMARY TARGETS
- rectus abdominis
- transversus abdominis

BENEFITS
- Abdominals
- Glutes
- Hamstrings
- Shoulders

CAUTIONS
- Avoid bouncing excessively and using momentum.

PERFECT YOUR FORM
- Keep your back flat throughout the movement.

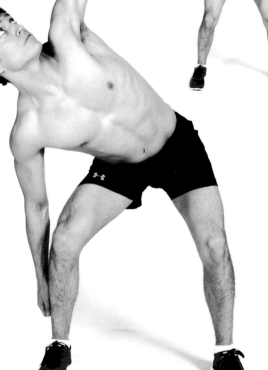

deltoideus anterior

deltoideus medialis

rectus abdominis

transversus abdominis*

SKIER

ADVANCED

THIS CORE EXERCISE focuses primarily on maintaining strength and control throughout a twisting motion. Your shoulder endurance will also come into play during this one as you concentrate on maintaining a stable upper body during a very dynamic lower body and hip movement. Keep the movement controlled—an easier variation of the routine is to rotate to one side only.

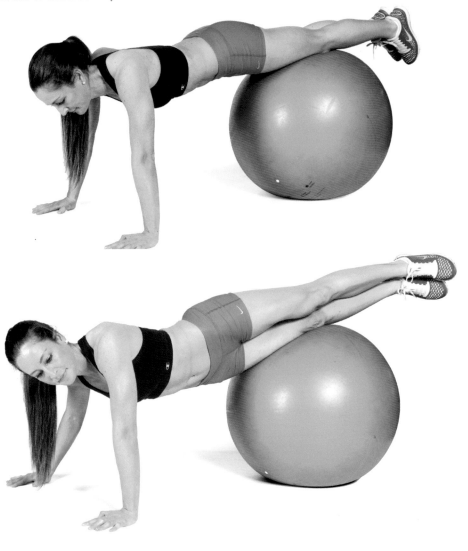

HOW TO DO IT

1 Begin in a push-up position, with your legs resting on a Swiss ball.

2 While maintaining your core position, rotate your trunk quickly to the left so that your legs are stacked on top of each other.

3 Return to the starting position, and perform the same movement to the right. Complete 15 full rotations.

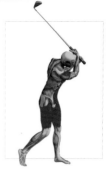

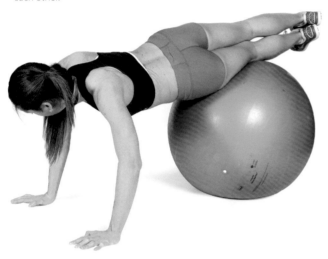

PRIMARY TARGETS

- sartorius
- iliopsoas
- iliacus
- tensor fasciae latae
- tractus iliotibialis
- rectus abdominis
- transversus abdominis
- multifidus spinae
- obliquus externus
- obliquus internus

BENEFITS

- Hips
- Core
- Upper back
- Posterior deltoids

CAUTIONS

- Avoid excessive speed.

PERFECT YOUR FORM

- Keep a tight core throughout the movement.

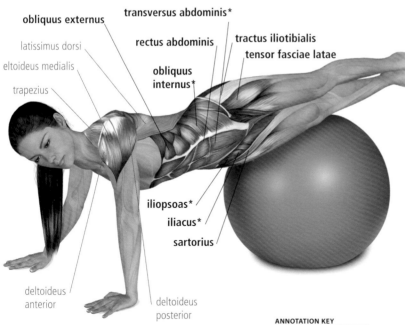

obliquus externus

transversus abdominis*

latissimus dorsi

rectus abdominis

tractus iliotibialis

eltoideus medialis

tensor fasciae latae

trapezius

obliquus internus*

iliopsoas*

iliacus*

sartorius

deltoideus anterior

deltoideus posterior

ANNOTATION KEY

Black text indicates strengthening muscles
Gray text indicates stretching muscles
Italic text indicates tendons and ligaments
- - - - *indicates deep muscles

MEDICINE BALL WOODCHOP

BEGINNER

ANOTHER STRAIGHTFORWARD routine using a medicine ball, the Medicine Ball Woodchop targets the obliques, rectus abdominis and erectors. Its principal benefit is to strengthen the obliques.

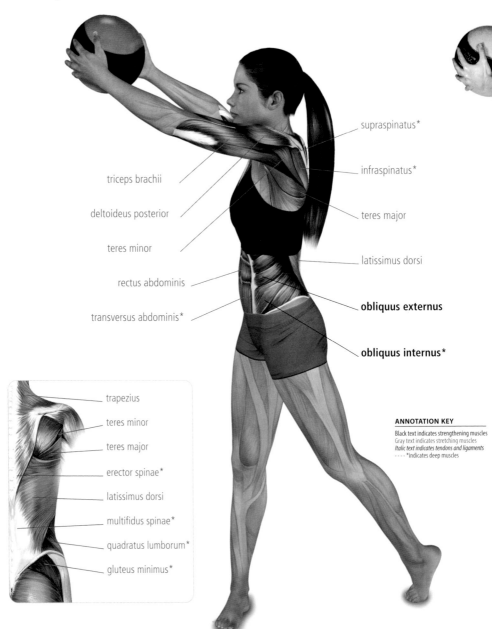

supraspinatus*

infraspinatus*

triceps brachii

teres major

deltoideus posterior

latissimus dorsi

teres minor

rectus abdominis

obliquus externus

transversus abdominis*

obliquus internus*

trapezius

teres minor

teres major

erector spinae*

latissimus dorsi

multifidus spinae*

quadratus lumborum*

gluteus minimus*

ANNOTATION KEY

Black text indicates strengthening muscles
Gray text indicates stretching muscles
Italic text indicates tendons and ligaments
- - - - *indicates deep muscles

HOW TO DO IT

1 Stand upright, with your feet shoulder-width apart, holding a medicine ball with both hands to the right side of your head.

2 Twist your core toward the left while lowering the medicine ball to the outside of your left leg, then return to the starting position. Repeat 20 times, then switch to the other side.

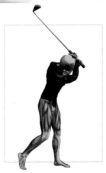

PRIMARY TARGETS
- obliquus externus
- obliquus internus

BENEFITS
- Obliques
- Rectus abdominis
- Erectors

CAUTIONS
- Avoid twisting too violently from side to side, since this can throw your back out.

PERFECT YOUR FORM
- Perform the positive portion of the exercise (swinging) aggressively and the negative portion (the wind-up) in a slow, controlled fashion, all the while keeping your core contracted and tight.

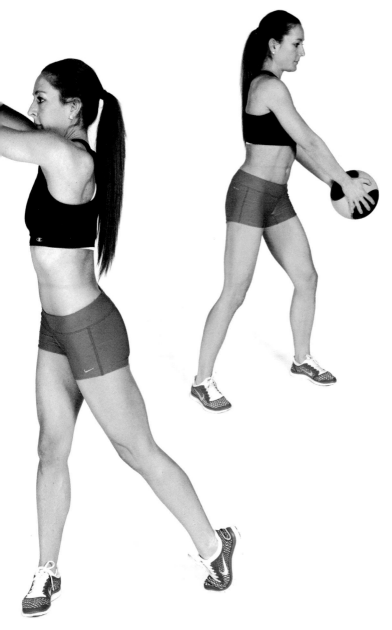

SWISS BALL JACK KNIFE

ADVANCED

THE SWISS BALL JACKKNIFE is a strength builder—primarily in the trunk and hips. For proper performance, you need to use coordination, timing, accuracy and strength.

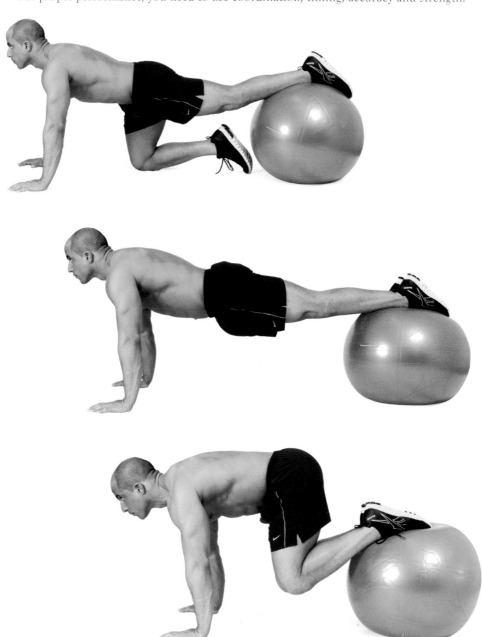

HOW TO DO IT

1 Kneel on your hands and knees, with the Swiss ball behind you. Your hands should be planted on the floor, with your arms straight.

2 One at a time, place your feet on the ball so that your legs are fully extended behind you and your body forms a line from head to toe. Find your balance.

3 Flex your hips, and pull your knees toward your chest, driving your hips toward the ceiling and retracting your abdomen.

4 Continuing to engage your abs, pull the ball further toward you. Maintain form in your upper body as you raise your buttocks toward the ceiling.

5 Hold for 5 seconds. Then, straighten your legs to the starting position. Begin with 10 repetitions, working up to 20.

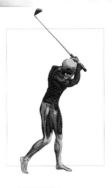

PRIMARY TARGETS
- rectus abdominis
- rectus femoris
- tensor fasciae latae
- Iliopsoas*
- pectineus*

BENEFITS
- Improves coordination
- Strengthens core

CAUTIONS
- Avoid arching your back or neck.

PERFECT YOUR FORM
- Engage your core, keeping your abs pulled inward.

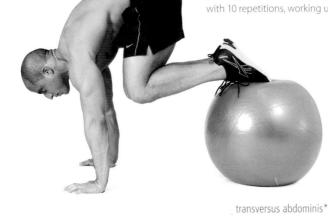

obliquus externus
obliquus internus*
erector spinae*
rhomboideus*
latissimus dorsi
teres major
transversus abdominis*
Iliopsoas*
tensor fasciae latae
rectus abdominis
pectoralis major
pectoralis minor*
deltoideus posterior
triceps brachii
tibialis anterior
rectus femoris
flexor carpi ulnaris

ANNOTATION KEY

Black text indicates strengthening muscles
Gray text indicates stretching muscles
Italic text indicates tendons and ligaments
----*indicates deep muscles

PUSH-UP WALKOUT

INTERMEDIATE

THE PUSH-UP WALKOUT is an excellent exercise for upper body and core strength. Push-up walkouts can be done at home or in the gym—they work the chest, triceps, shoulders and core.

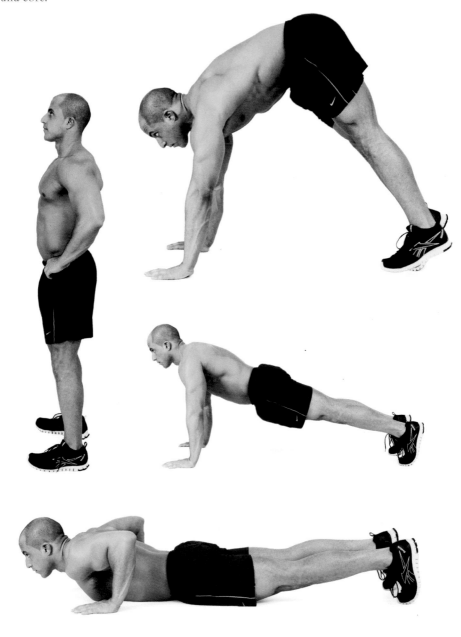

HOW TO DO IT

1 Stand with your feet hip-width apart.

2 Bend forward until your hands reach the floor.

3 'Walk' your hands out in front of you as far as possible.

4 Press your palms into the floor and tuck your toes so that you are in an upper push-up position. Perform a push-up.

5 'Walk' the hands back toward your feet. Roll back up to starting position.

6 Work up to 10 repetitions.

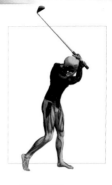

PRIMARY TARGETS
- rectus abdominis
- transversus abdominis*
- latissimus dorsi
- pectoralis major
- brachialis
- coracobrachialis*
- pectoralis minor*
- deltoideus anterior

BENEFITS
- Strengthens and tones core, chest and back muscles

CAUTIONS
- Avoid arching your back or hunching forward.

PERFECT YOUR FORM
- Keep your feet planted on the floor as you 'walk' your hands forward and back.

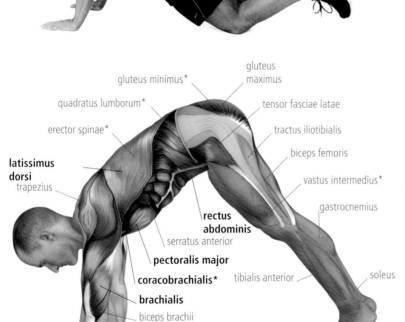

gluteus minimus*

gluteus maximus

quadratus lumborum*

tensor fasciae latae

erector spinae*

tractus iliotibialis

latissimus dorsi

biceps femoris

trapezius

vastus intermedius*

gastrocnemius

rectus abdominis

serratus anterior

pectoralis major

tibialis anterior

soleus

coracobrachialis*

brachialis

biceps brachii

ANNOTATION KEY

Black text indicates strengthening muscles
Gray text indicates stretching muscles
Italic text indicates tendons and ligaments
- - - - *indicates deep muscles

ARM-REACH PLANK

ADVANCED

THE ARM-REACH PLANK is a conditioning routine that focuses on the rectus abdominis, erector spinae, and oblique muscles. It is excellent for strengthening the entire core. For a greater challenge, lift one foot off the floor while carrying out the exercise.

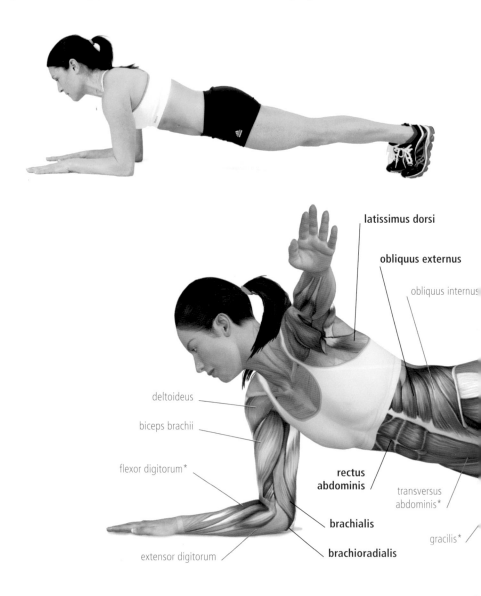

latissimus dorsi

obliquus externus

obliquus internus

deltoideus

biceps brachii

flexor digitorum*

rectus abdominis

transversus abdominis*

brachialis

gracilis*

extensor digitorum

brachioradialis

HOW TO DO IT

1 Begin face-down, resting on your forearms and knees.

2 One at a time, step your feet back into a plank position. Engage your abdominal muscles and find a neutral spine.

3 Maintaining proper plank form, slowly lift your right arm off the floor. Hold for 30 seconds. Release and return to starting position.

4 Switch arms and repeat. Aim to hold for 60 seconds as you become stronger.

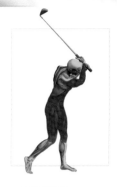

PRIMARY TARGETS
- brachioradialis
- brachialis
- latissimus dorsi
- rectus abdominis
- obliquus externus
- tractus iliotibialis
- rectus femoris

BENEFITS
- Improves balance
- Strengthens and tones arms, legs and abdominal muscles

CAUTIONS
- Avoid allowing your hips to sink or tilt upward.

PERFECT YOUR FORM
- Contract your abdominal muscles.

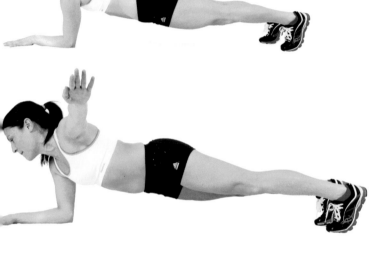

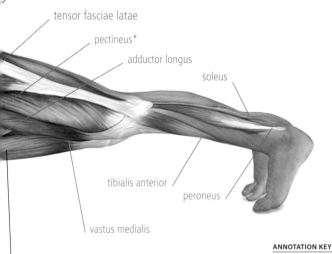

tractus iliotibialis

tensor fasciae latae

pectineus*

adductor longus

soleus

tibialis anterior

peroneus

vastus medialis

rectus femoris

ANNOTATION KEY

Black text indicates strengthening muscles
Gray text indicates stretching muscles
Italic text indicates tendons and ligaments
- - - - *indicates deep muscles

TWISTING KNEE RAISE

INTERMEDIATE

THE TWISTING KNEE RAISE is a strength builder, primarily of the trunk and calves. Strength, coordination and timing are required to perform this exercise correctly. The routine is slow-paced and is performed for longer amounts of time than most exercises—in doing so it helps to develop "slow strength" and muscular endurance rather than explosive power or speed.

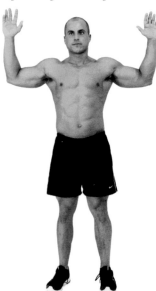

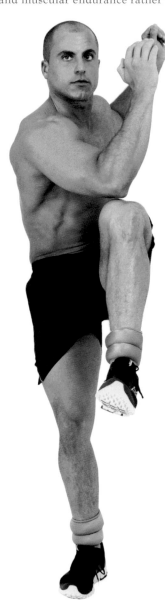

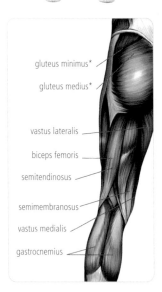

gluteus minimus*

gluteus medius*

vastus lateralis

biceps femoris

semitendinosus

semimembranosus

vastus medialis

gastrocnemius

HOW TO DO IT

1 Stand with your feet hip-width apart and your arms at your sides. Raise both arms and bend your elbows so that each arm forms a right angle, palms facing forward.

2 Raise your left knee toward your abdomen. At the same time, bring your right elbow toward the knee. Aim for your knee and elbow to touch.

3 Return to starting position. Repeat, alternating sides. Aim for 20 repetitions.

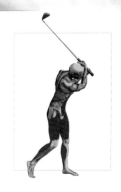

PRIMARY TARGETS
- extensor carpi radialis
- extensor carpi ulnaris
- extensor digiti minimi
- extensor digitorum
- extensor indicis
- extensor pollicis

BENEFITS
- Wrists
- Hands
- Forearms

CAUTIONS
- Avoid lifting or tensing your shoulders.

PERFECT YOUR FORM
- Be sure to press your thumb into the meaty part of your palm, attached to the thumb, intensifying the stretch in your forearm and wrist.

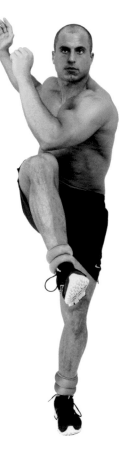

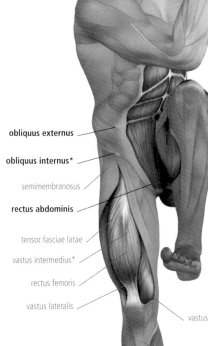

obliquus externus

obliquus internus*

semimembranosus

rectus abdominis

tensor fasciae latae

vastus intermedius*

rectus femoris

vastus lateralis

vastus medialis

gastrocnemius

ANNOTATION KEY

Black text indicates strengthening muscles
Gray text indicates stretching muscles
Italic text indicates tendons and ligaments
- - - - *indicates deep muscles

TWISTING LIFT

INTERMEDIATE

THE TWISTING LIFT is a great exercise for building endurance and also strengthens and tones your arms while working your obliques. Be sure to keep the movement smooth and at an even speed.

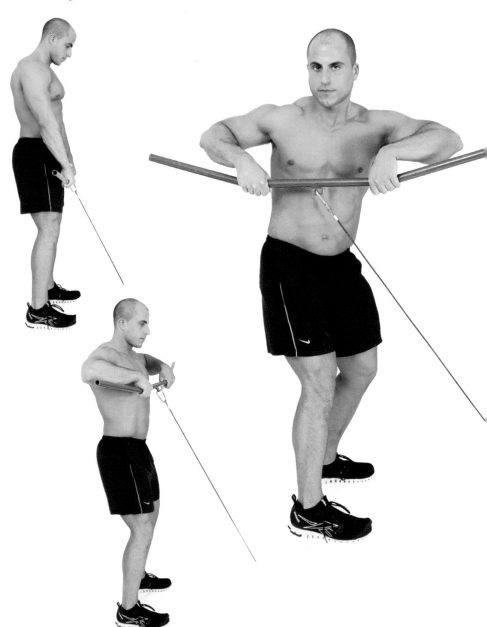

HOW TO DO IT

1 Stand upright, facing a cable machine, with your feet planted hip-distance apart or slightly wider. Hold the cable in both hands.

2 In a smooth movement, pull the cable toward your body as you bend your elbows to bring the cable in toward your chest. Your elbows should be almost at shoulder height.

3 Using your hips as a hinge, turn to the right side. Your arms should stay in place. Allow your left knee to bend slightly if desired.

4 Gradually twist back to starting position, facing the machine.

5 Straighten your arms, releasing the cable to return to starting position. Switch sides and repeat, aiming for 20 per side.

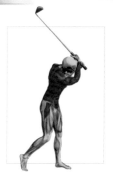

PRIMARY TARGETS
• trapezius
• deltoideus medialis
• rectus abdominis
• obliquus externus
• obliquus internus*

BENEFITS
• Strengthens and tones arms and oblique muscles

CAUTIONS
• Avoid moving in a jerky manner.

PERFECT YOUR FORM
• Keep your feet planted and your torso stable as you move.

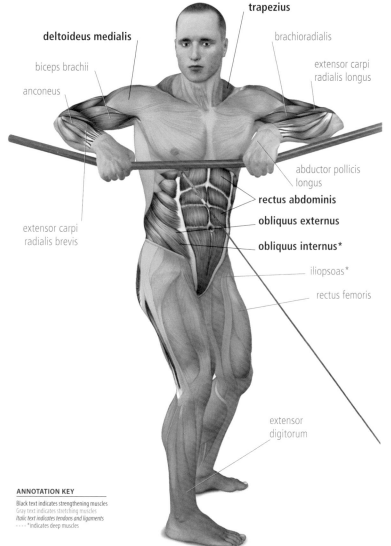

trapezius

deltoideus medialis

biceps brachii

anconeus

brachioradialis

extensor carpi radialis longus

abductor pollicis longus

rectus abdominis

obliquus externus

obliquus internus*

iliopsoas*

rectus femoris

extensor carpi radialis brevis

extensor digitorum

ANNOTATION KEY
Black text indicates strengthening muscles
Gray text indicates stretching muscles
Italic text indicates tendons and ligaments
- - - -*indicates deep muscles

CROSSOVER CRUNCH

INTERMEDIATE

THE CROSSOVER CRUNCH is a great exercise because it not only targets the abdominal muscles but also the oblique muscles, which run along the side of your ribcage. This makes it a great exercise if you are looking for a total core workout. It can also help stabilize your back, thereby reducing and preventing back pain and spasms.

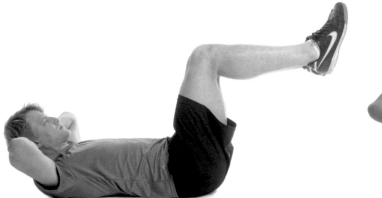

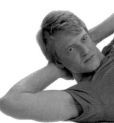

biceps brachii

deltoideus anterior

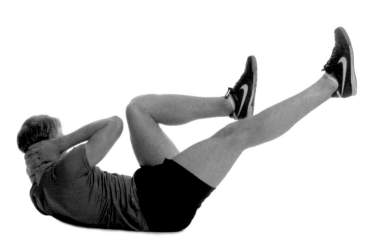

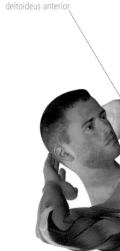

latissimus dorsi

serratus anterior

rectus abdominis

HOW TO DO IT

1 Bring your hands behind your head, and lift your legs off the floor into a tabletop position, so that your thighs and calves form a 90-degree angle.

2 Roll up with your torso, reaching your right elbow to your left knee and extending the right leg in front of you. Imagine pulling your shoulder blades off the floor and twisting from your ribs and oblique muscles.

3 Alternate sides. Repeat sequence six times.

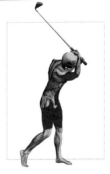

PRIMARY TARGETS
- ectus abdominis
- transversus abdominis
- obliquus externus
- obliquus internus

BENEFITS
- Torso stabilisers
- Abdominals

CAUTIONS
- Avoid pulling with your hands.
- Bringing your chin toward your chest.
- Arching your back.
- Moving the active elbow faster than your shoulder.

PERFECT YOUR FORM
- Elongate your neck.
- Lift your chin away from your chest.
- Keep both hips stable on the floor.

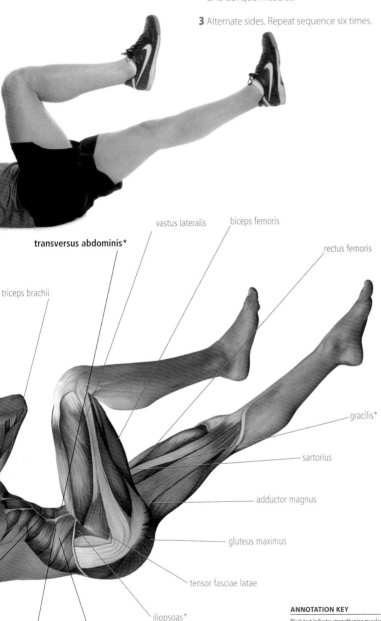

transversus abdominis*

vastus lateralis

biceps femoris

rectus femoris

triceps brachii

gracilis*

sartorius

adductor magnus

gluteus maximus

tensor fasciae latae

iliopsoas*

bliquus externus

obliquus internus*

ANNOTATION KEY

Black text indicates strengthening muscles
Gray text indicates stretching muscles
Italic text indicates tendons and ligaments
- - - - *indicates deep muscles

DIAGONAL REACH

INTERMEDIATE

THE DIAGONAL REACH is a simple but effective exercise that can be made more difficult by reaching further, bringing your arms to a steeper diagonal in one direction while raising the opposite foot off the floor.

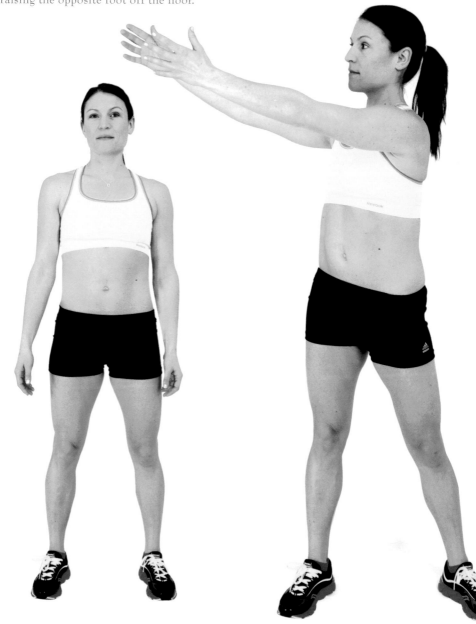

HOW TO DO IT

1 Stand with your feet hip-width apart and your arms at your sides.

2 Raise both arms upward and to the right to form a diagonal line. Follow

your hands with your gaze. Return to starting position.

3 Repeat to the left side. Perform 12 repetitions.

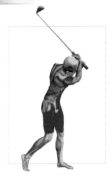

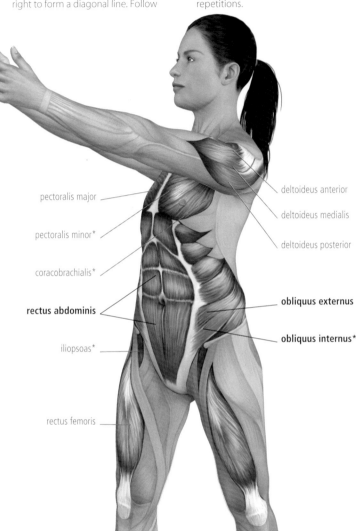

pectoralis major

pectoralis minor*

coracobrachialis*

rectus abdominis

iliopsoas*

rectus femoris

deltoideus anterior

deltoideus medialis

deltoideus posterior

obliquus externus

obliquus internus*

PRIMARY TARGETS
- rectus abdominis
- obliquus internus*
- obliquus externus

BENEFITS
- Stretches and strengthens the muscles used for twisting

CAUTIONS
- Avoid twisting your hips.
- Tensing your neck as you lift or lower your arms.

PERFECT YOUR FORM
- Keep your abdominal muscles engaged.
- Keep your hips facing forward.

ANNOTATION KEY
Black text indicates strengthening muscles
Gray text indicates stretching muscles
Italic text indicates tendons and ligaments
- - - - *indicates deep muscles

LEG EXTENSION CHAIR DIP

INTERMEDIATE

THE LEG EXTENSION CHAIR DIP is a good exercise for both the triceps muscles and the quadriceps in the raised leg. It also works the core muscles, which need to be engaged as you perform the exercise.

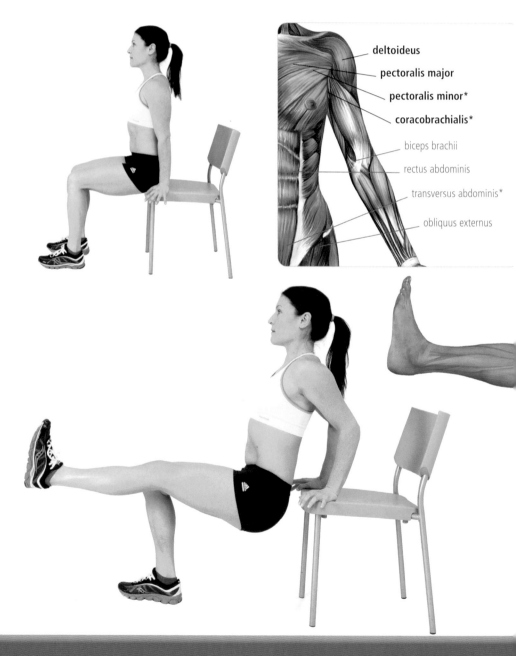

deltoideus

pectoralis major

pectoralis minor*

coracobrachialis*

biceps brachii

rectus abdominis

transversus abdominis*

obliquus externus

HOW TO DO IT

1 Sit on the very edge of a chair, with your palms on the seat. Your back should be straight, your knees bent to form 90-degree angles.

2 Slowly and with control, engage your abdominal muscles and press your palms into the seat as you move your buttocks forward and lower slightly so that you are no longer resting on the chair.

3 Bending your arms slightly, extend your left leg forward to form a straight line.

4 Return your foot to the floor. Repeat on the other side, working up to 10 repetitions per side. Release and return to starting position.

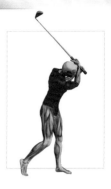

PRIMARY TARGETS
- pectoralis major
- pectoralis minor*
- coracobrachialis*
- deltoideus
- deltoideus

BENEFITS
- Improves balance
- Strengthens legs and triceps

CAUTIONS
- Avoid arching your back or hunching forward.

PERFECT YOUR FORM
- Keep your supporting foot anchored to the floor.

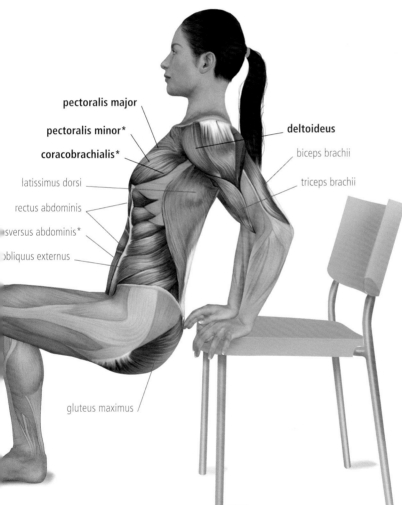

pectoralis major

pectoralis minor*

coracobrachialis*

latissimus dorsi

rectus abdominis

...sversus abdominis*

...obliquus externus

deltoideus

biceps brachii

triceps brachii

gluteus maximus

ANNOTATION KEY

Black text indicates strengthening muscles
Gray text indicates stretching muscles
Italic text indicates tendons and ligaments
- - - - *indicates deep muscles

PLANK

ADVANCED

THE PLANK EXERCISE is a great way to build endurance in both the abs and back, as well as strengthening the stabilizer muscles. This move is also great for building strength for pushups, an exercise that requires considerable core strength.

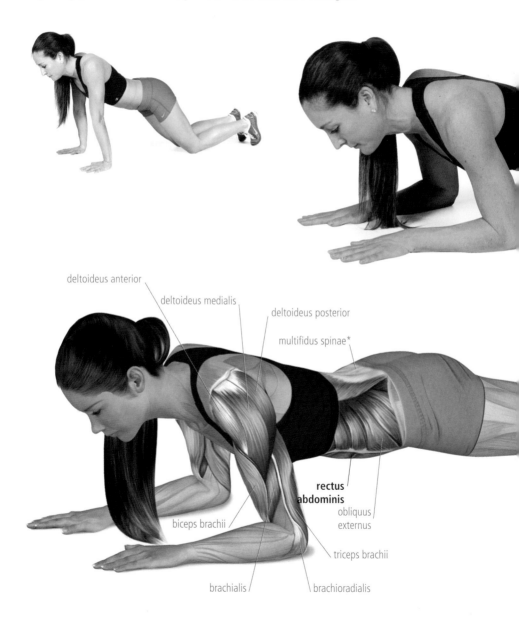

deltoideus anterior

deltoideus medialis

deltoideus posterior

multifidus spinae*

**rectus
abdominis**

obliquus
externus

biceps brachii

triceps brachii

brachialis

brachioradialis

HOW TO DO IT

1 Position yourself on all fours.

2 Plant your forearms on the floor parallel to one another, then raise your knees off the floor and lengthen your legs until they are in line with your arms.

3 Hold this plank position for 30 seconds (building up to 120 seconds).

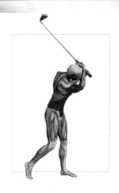

PRIMARY TARGETS
• Rectus abdominis
• Erector spinae
• Obliques

BENEFITS
• Strengthens the entire core

CAUTIONS
• Avoid bridging too high, since this can take stress off working muscles.

PERFECT YOUR FORM
• Keep your abdominal muscles tight and your body in a straight line.

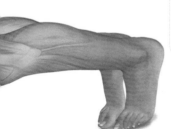

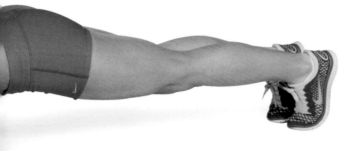

pectoralis major

serratus anterior

rectus abdominis

obliquus externus

obliquus internus*

transversus abdominis*

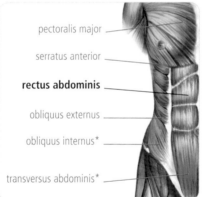

ANNOTATION KEY

Black text indicates strengthening muscles
Gray text indicates stretching muscles
Italic text indicates tendons and ligaments
- - - - *indicates deep muscles

WOODCHOP

ADVANCED

THERE ARE SEVERAL VERSIONS of the woodchop exercise: with a low-to-high motion, as illustrated here, high-to-low, and even kneeling with the opposite leg up. If you don't have access to a cable machine, you can use a medicine ball, kettlebell or a heavy plate.

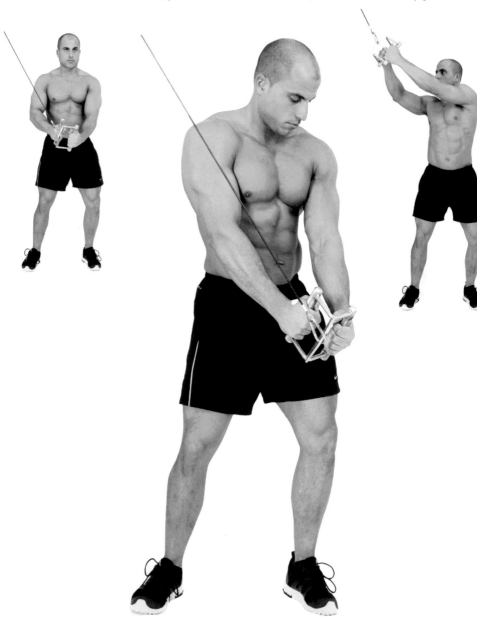

HOW TO DO IT

1 Stand with your feet slightly wider than hip-distance part, with each weight machine to your right. Grasp the handle of the cable in both hands. Your legs may be slightly bent.

2 Slowly and smoothly, rotate your core and raise your arms diagonally to the upper right, toward the cable machine.

3 In a controlled 'chopping' motion, bring your arms diagonally back to starting position and then down to the other side, rotating your core away from the machine.

4 Complete 10 repetitions. Then, switch sides and repeat.

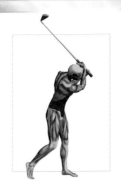

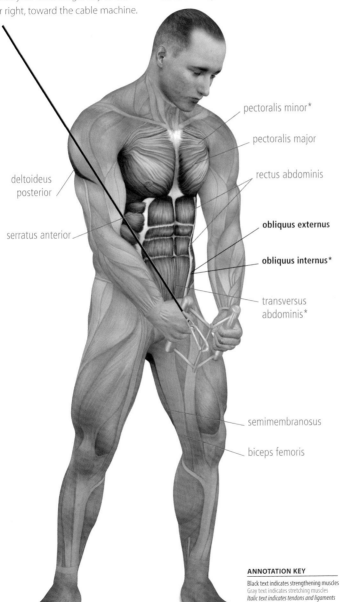

deltoideus posterior

serratus anterior

pectoralis minor*

pectoralis major

rectus abdominis

obliquus externus

obliquus internus*

transversus abdominis*

semimembranosus

biceps femoris

PRIMARY TARGETS
• obliquus externus
• obliquus internus*

BENEFITS
• Strengthens and tones arms and oblique muscles
• Builds endurance

CAUTIONS
• Avoid raising your arms so high that you lose control of your core and/or arch your back.

PERFECT YOUR FORM
• You can also perform this exercise with a resistance band, anchoring one end beneath one foot, holding the other end in both hands, and twisting in the opposite direction.

ANNOTATION KEY

Black text indicates strengthening muscles
Gray text indicates stretching muscles
Italic text indicates tendons and ligaments
- - - - *indicates deep muscles

KNEE-FLEXION BALL THROW

INTERMEDIATE

The Knee-Flexion Ball Throw requires a partner to perform effectively (or you'll be doing a lot of chasing and fetching—no bad thing if you have the space for it). It's primary function is to improve rotation ability and upper body range of motion.

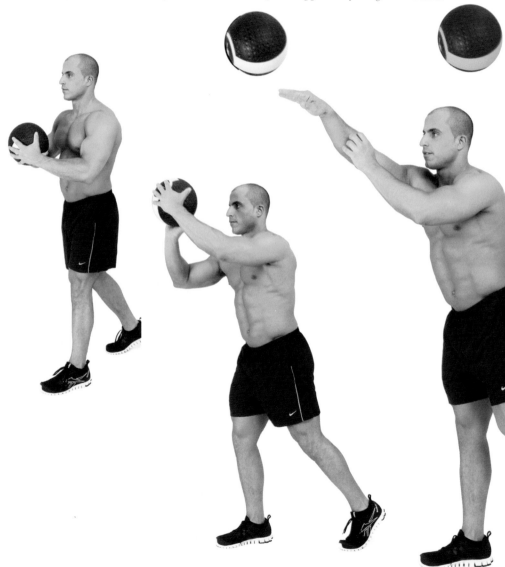

HOW TO DO IT

1 Hold a weighted medicine ball in front of your chest, taking a few steps forward to get ready if you choose.

2 Prepare to throw the ball by positioning your left foot behind you, heel off the floor. Keeping your torso stable, raise the ball until it is positioned above your right shoulder.

3 Bend the knee of your back foot to lift it off the ground as you throw the ball forward.

4 Retrieve the ball (or have someone toss it back to you). Then, repeat on the opposite side, performing 10 throws.

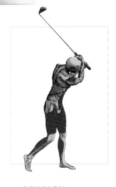

PRIMARY TARGETS
- rectus femoris
- vastus lateralis
- vastus intermedius*
- vastus medialis
- rectus abdominis
- gluteus maximus
- gluteus medius*
- gluteus minimus*
- obliquus internus*
- obliquus externus
- erector spinae*

BENEFITS
- Improves coordination, core rotational ability and range of motion in upper body
- Strengthens and stabilises core

CAUTIONS
- Avoid excessively twisting your torso to either side.

PERFECT YOUR FORM
- Engage your abdominal muscles as you throw.

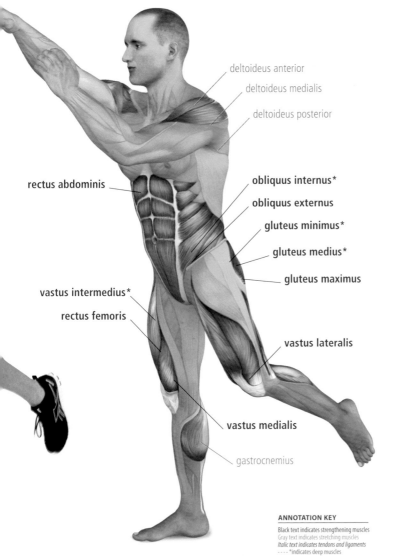

deltoideus anterior

deltoideus medialis

deltoideus posterior

rectus abdominis

obliquus internus*

obliquus externus

gluteus minimus*

gluteus medius*

gluteus maximus

vastus intermedius*

rectus femoris

vastus lateralis

vastus medialis

gastrocnemius

ANNOTATION KEY

Black text indicates strengthening muscles
Gray text indicates stretching muscles
Italic text indicates tendons and ligaments
- - - - *indicates deep muscles

FIGURE 8

ADVANCED

THE FIGURE 8 is a simple but comprehensive routine that targets a wide range of muscles, including those in the shoulders, core, thighs, upper back, glutes and triceps. It increases stability in the hips and aids balance throughout the body.

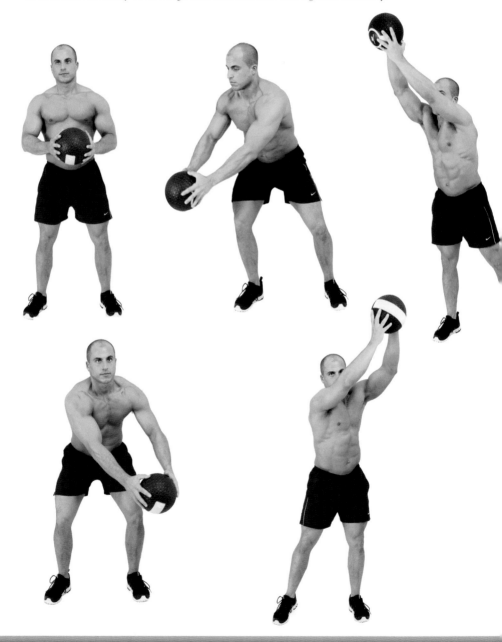

HOW TO DO IT

1 Stand with your feet hip-width apart or slightly wider. Grasp a medicine ball in both hands, and hold it in front of your torso.

2 Shift your weight to the right. In a smooth, controlled movement, extend both arms and bring the medicine ball toward the lower right side of your body.

3 Continue shifting your weight to the right, bringing the right heel off the floor if desired as you raise the ball toward the upper right side of your body.

4 In a Figure 8 motion, bring the ball diagonally toward the lower left side of your body, and then raise it to the upper left as you shift your weight onto your left leg.

5 Repeat 5 times in this direction. Then, switch directions and repeat.

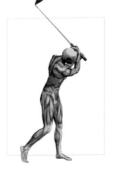

PRIMARY TARGETS
• rectus abdominis
• obliquus externus
• obliquus internus*
• biceps femoris

BENEFITS
• Improves coordination, flexibility and range of motion
• Strengthens and tones core and arm muscles

CAUTIONS
• Avoid straining your neck.
• Avoid tensing or hunching your shoulders.

PERFECT YOUR FORM
• Keep your core muscles engaged and your abs pulled inward.

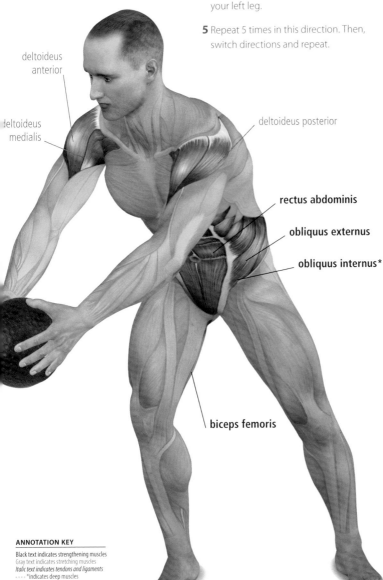

deltoideus anterior

deltoideus medialis

deltoideus posterior

rectus abdominis

obliquus externus

obliquus internus*

biceps femoris

ANNOTATION KEY

Black text indicates strengthening muscles
Gray text indicates stretching muscles
Italic text indicates tendons and ligaments
- - - - *indicates deep muscles

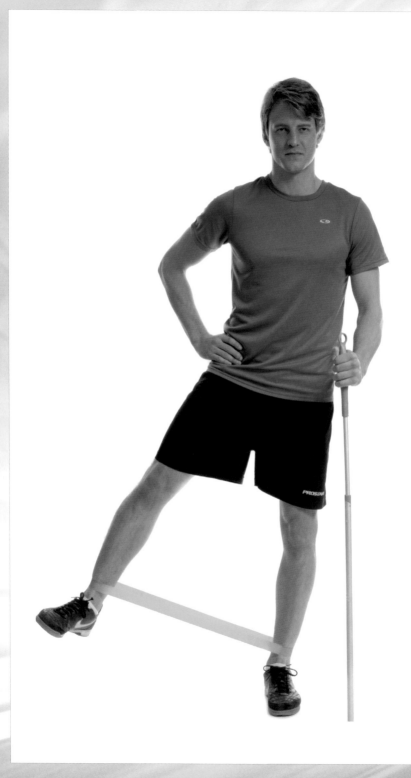

GLUTES

The hip muscles, specifically the glutes, help contribute to a strong base and will contribute to knee stability by controlling femoral motion. They are important for developing force during the downswing. Your glutes, in addition to your ankles, also play a large role with balance, especially if you are on an uneven surface. The main components of your program should be stabilization, strengthening and then power development. In terms of golf-specific training, many of the best exercises will mimic the motions performed in the sport, which is a large part of the thinking behind the exercises selected here.

PIGEON STRETCH

STRETCH

THE PIGEON STRETCH promotes myofascial release in the glutes, stretching the gluteus maximus and the gluteus medius and minimus muscles above it.

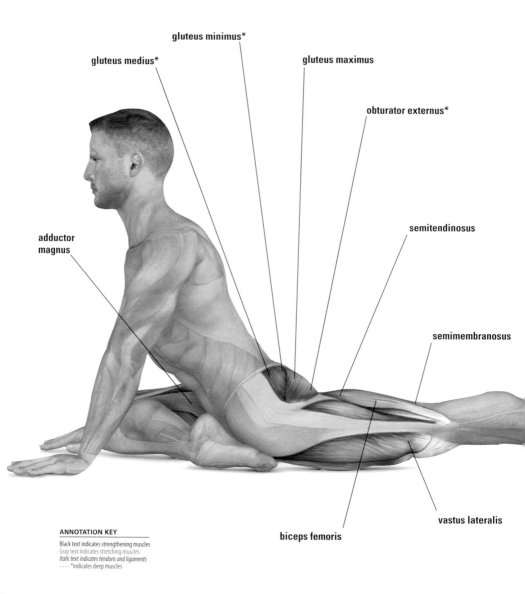

gluteus minimus*

gluteus medius*

gluteus maximus

obturator externus*

semitendinosus

adductor magnus

semimembranosus

vastus lateralis

biceps femoris

ANNOTATION KEY
Black text indicates strengthening muscles
Gray text indicates stretching muscles
Italic text indicates tendons and ligaments
---- *indicates deep muscles

HOW TO DO IT

1 Kneel with your buttocks resting lightly on your heels and your arms at your sides, supporting some of your weight.

2 Straighten your left leg to extend it along the floor behind you, keeping the leg in parallel, aligned with your body, including your right knee, which should be facing straight forward.

3 Move your arms forward to rest slightly in front of your right knee. Your hands should be shoulder-width apart and flat on the floor, palms down.

4 Keeping the rest of your body in alignment, move your right heel a few inches to the left so that it crosses the core of your body.

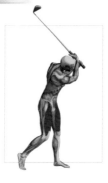

PRIMARY TARGETS

- adductor longus
- adductor magnus
- adductor brevis
- gracilis
- pectineus
- obturator externus
- rectus femoris
- vastus lateralis
- vastus intermedius
- vastus medialis
- biceps femoris
- semitendinosus
- semimembranosus
- gluteus maximus
- gluteus medius
- gluteus minimus
- iliopsoas

BENEFITS

- Gluteal area
- Groin muscles
- Hamstrings
- Quadriceps

CAUTIONS

- Avoid hyperextending your elbows.

PERFECT YOUR FORM

- Maintain a slight bend in your elbows.
- Lean primarily on your bent leg.

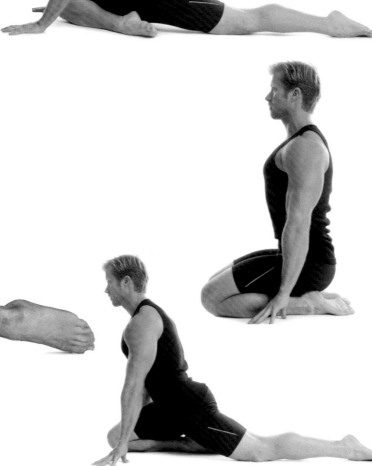

LYING-DOWN FIGURE 4

STRETCH

THE FIGURE 4 improves malleability of the main muscle in the buttocks, the gluteus maximus, as well as the smaller gluteus medius and gluteus minimus. These are some of the most important muscles in the body for mobility, so it is vital to keep them stretched and flexible.

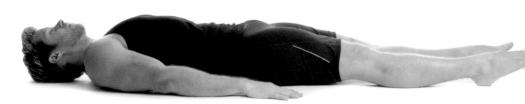

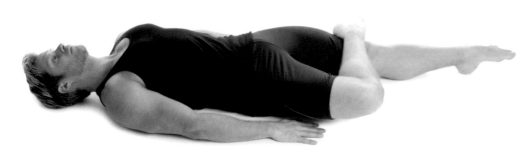

ANNOTATION KEY

Black text indicates strengthening muscles
Gray text indicates stretching muscles
Italic text indicates tendons and ligaments
- - - - *indicates deep muscles

HOW TO DO IT

1 Lie on your back with your legs extended.

2 Point both toes. Bend your right knee and turn the leg out so that your right ankle rests on your left thigh just above the knee, creating a figure 4.

3 Bend your left leg, drawing both legs (still in the figure 4 position) in toward your chest as you grasp the back of your left thigh.

4 Push your right elbow against your right inner thigh, turning out the right leg slightly to increase the intensity of the stretch.

5 Return to the starting position, switch legs, and repeat.

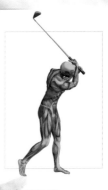

PRIMARY TARGETS
- gluteus maximus
- gluteus medius
- gluteus minimus
- piriformis

BENEFITS
- Gluteal region

CAUTIONS
- Keep your head and shoulder blades on the floor.

PERFECT YOUR FORM
- Be sure to press your thumb into the meaty part of your palm, attached to the thumb, intensifying the stretch in your forearm and wrist.

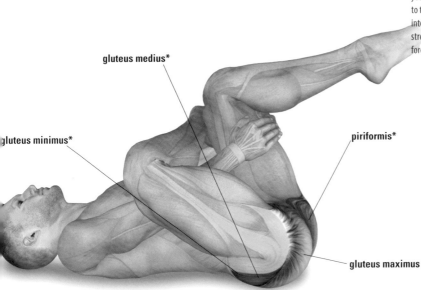

gluteus medius*

gluteus minimus*

piriformis*

gluteus maximus

SEATED LEG CRADLE

STRETCH

THE SEATED LEG CRADLE (or "Baby Cradle Pose" as it is called in yoga) is a great hip opening exercise that beginners can perform with the aid of a blanket or block. It is a great stretch for your glutes and upper hamstrings.

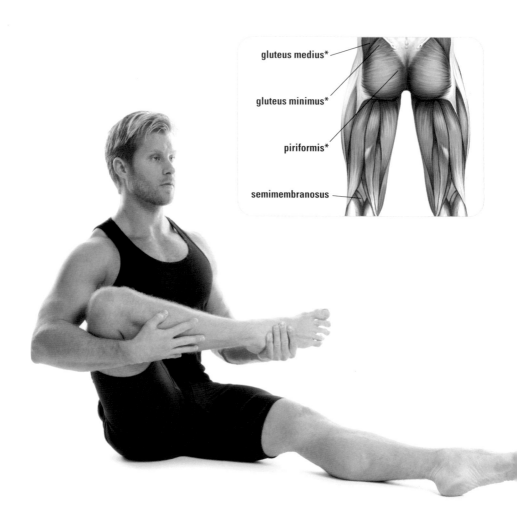

gluteus medius*

gluteus minimus*

piriformis*

semimembranosus

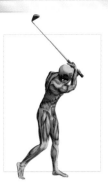

HOW TO DO IT

1 Sit on the floor with your legs extended in front of you.

2 Bend your right knee and grasp your calf with your right hand. With your left hand, support the raised foot as you hug it into your chest as if you were cradling a baby. Keep your heel roughly 12 inches away from your chest.

3 Switch sides, and repeat on the other leg.

PRIMARY TARGETS

- biceps femoris
- semitendinosus
- semimembranosus
- gluteus maximus
- gluteus medius
- gluteus minimus
- piriformis

BENEFITS

- Upper hamstrings
- Gluteal region

CAUTIONS

- Avoid holding your breath.

PERFECT YOUR FORM

- Keep your chest lifted.
- Contract your gluteal muscles.

ANNOTATION KEY

Black text indicates strengthening muscles
Gray text indicates stretching muscles
Italic text indicates tendons and ligaments
- - - - *indicates deep muscles

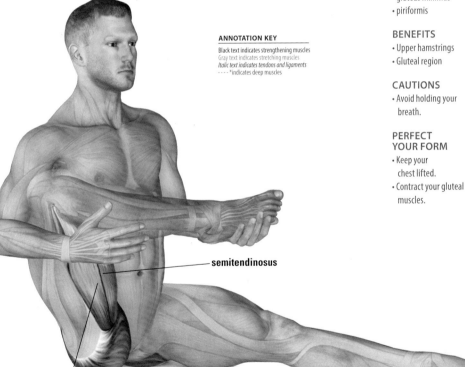

semitendinosus

gluteus maximus

biceps femoris

HIP EXTENSION WITH BAND

INTERMEDIATE

THE HIP EXTENSION WITH BAND focuses on your glutes and hamstrings. In particular, it builds strength in the three muscles that make up the glutes—the gluteus minimus, medius and maximus.

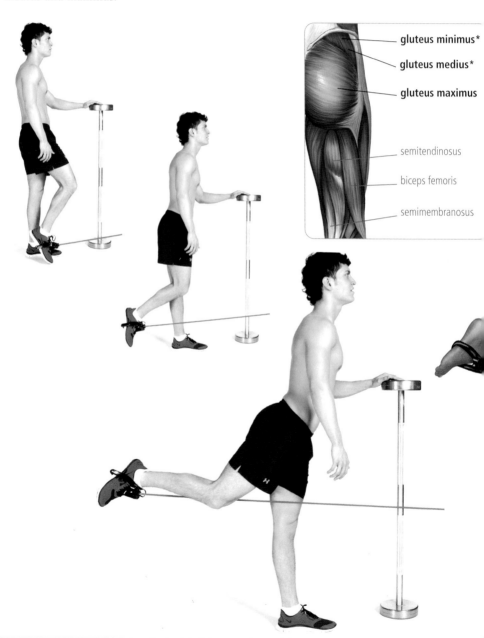

gluteus minimus*

gluteus medius*

gluteus maximus

semitendinosus

biceps femoris

semimembranosus

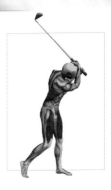

HOW TO DO IT

1 Loop one end of a band to the lower part of a post, and wrap the other end around your right ankle or foot.

2 Stand facing the post, holding a sturdy surface for support.

3 Maintaining an upright posture, extend the right leg as far back as you are able while also keeping it as straight as possible. Complete 10–12 repetitions, then switch legs.

PRIMARY TARGETS
- gluteus minimus
- gluteus medius
- gluteus maximus

BENEFITS
- Glutes
- Hamstrings

CAUTIONS
- Avoid an excessive kicking motion.

PERFECT YOUR FORM
- Maintain an upright posture throughout the movement.

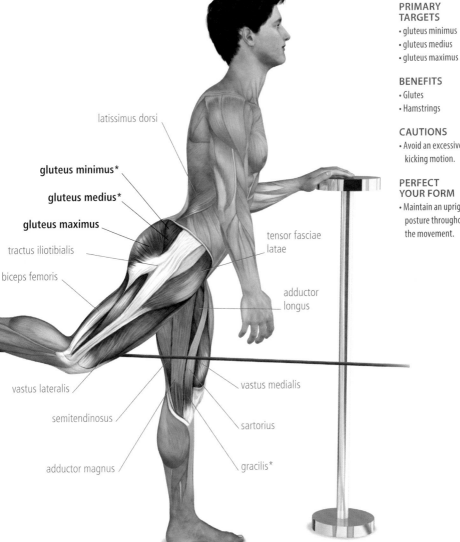

latissimus dorsi

gluteus minimus*

gluteus medius*

gluteus maximus

tractus iliotibialis

biceps femoris

tensor fasciae latae

adductor longus

vastus lateralis

vastus medialis

semitendinosus

sartorius

adductor magnus

gracilis*

ANNOTATION KEY

Black text indicates strengthening muscles
Gray text indicates stretching muscles
Italic text indicates tendons and ligaments
- - - - *indicates deep muscles

LATERAL BOUNDING

BEGINNER

LATERAL BOUNDING TARGETS several areas, including the quadriceps, hamstrings, glutes and calves. Its principal aim is to help you practice lateral movement at speed. Try completing a set of jumps to one side, and then switching. Alternatively, add an extra level of difficulty by performing the routine while holding a medicine ball.

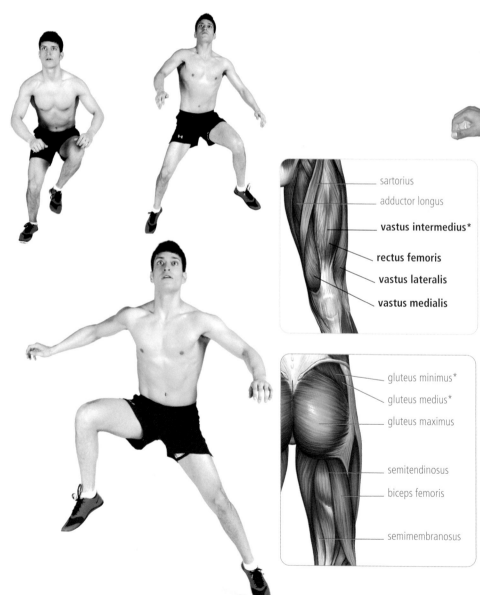

sartorius

adductor longus

vastus intermedius*

rectus femoris

vastus lateralis

vastus medialis

gluteus minimus*

gluteus medius*

gluteus maximus

semitendinosus

biceps femoris

semimembranosus

HOW TO DO IT

1 Start in a quarter-squat position, then bound off your right foot as far and high as possible to your left.

2 Be sure to land on your left foot.

3 Next, bound as far and as high as possible back to your right off your left foot. Perform 15 repetitions per side.

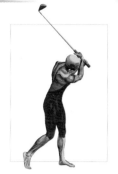

PRIMARY TARGETS
- vastus intermedius
- vastus lateralis
- vastus medialis
- rectus femoris

BENEFITS
- Quadriceps
- Hamstrings
- Glutes
- Calves

CAUTIONS
- Avoid allowing your knees to protrude past your toes.

PERFECT YOUR FORM
- Be sure to keep a tight core throughout the movement.

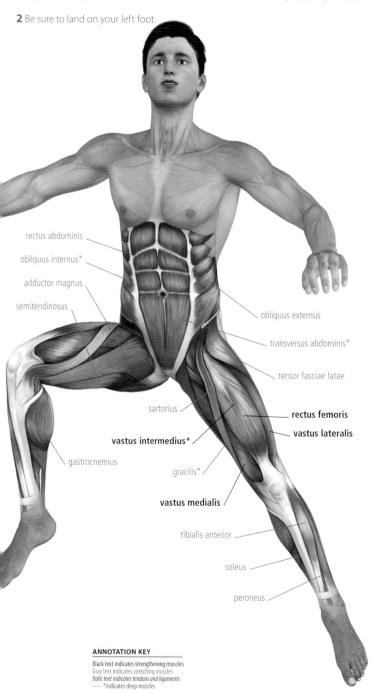

rectus abdominis

obliquus internus*

adductor magnus

semitendinosus

obliquus externus

transversus abdominis*

tensor fasciae latae

sartorius

rectus femoris

vastus lateralis

vastus intermedius*

gastrocnemius

gracilis*

vastus medialis

tibialis anterior

soleus

peroneus

ANNOTATION KEY

Black text indicates strengthening muscles
Gray text indicates stretching muscles
Italic text indicates tendons and ligaments
- - - - *indicates deep muscles

HEEL BEATS

ADVANCED

HEEL BEATS ARE an effective Pilates movement that engage the abdominals, inner thighs and glutes to help shape and create firm buttocks. It is one of the best glute exercises you can do on the mat. The main thing you have to remember is to keep your abdominal muscles pulled in and to go for length along your back and down the back of your legs so that you protect your lower back.

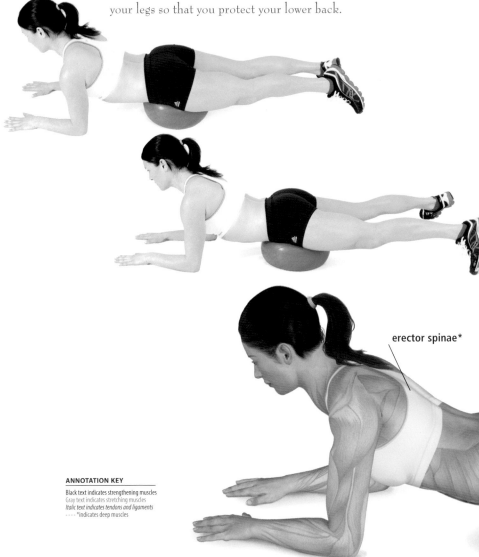

erector spinae*

ANNOTATION KEY
Black text indicates strengthening muscles
Gray text indicates stretching muscles
Italic text indicates tendons and ligaments
- - - - *indicates deep muscles

HOW TO DO IT

1 Lie facedown with your forearms on the floor. Rest your hips on top of a small Swiss ball. Extend your legs behind you.

2 Turn your legs out from the top of your hips.

3 Pull your navel up toward your spine, pressing your pubic bone into the ball. Lengthen your legs and lift them off the mat.

4 Press your heels together and then separate them in a rapid but controlled motion.

5 Beat your heels together for 8 counts. Release and then repeat, performing 6 repetitions.

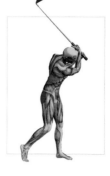

PRIMARY TARGETS
- gluteus maximus
- gluteus medius*
- gluteus minimus*
- erector spinae*
- sartorius
- pectineus*
- iliopsoas*

BENEFITS
- Stabilises core
- Tones abdominal muscles
- Improves coordination

CAUTIONS
- Avoid hunching your shoulders.

PERFECT YOUR FORM
- Press your shoulders down toward your back.

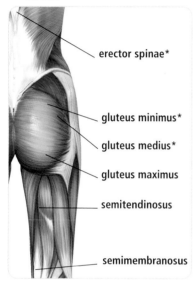

erector spinae*

gluteus minimus*

gluteus medius*

gluteus maximus

semitendinosus

semimembranosus

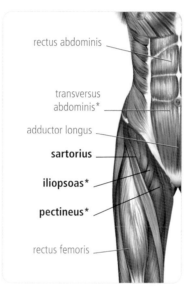

rectus abdominis

transversus abdominis*

adductor longus

sartorius

iliopsoas*

pectineus*

rectus femoris

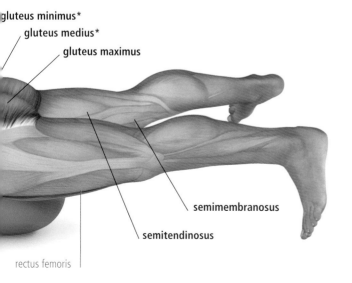

gluteus minimus*

gluteus medius*

gluteus maximus

semimembranosus

semitendinosus

rectus femoris

PIRIFORMIS BRIDGE

BEGINNER

As with many functional exercises, the Piriformis Bridge combines two classic exercises into one—in this instance the combination is the Piriformis (or Supine) Stretch and the classic Bridge. The result is an exercise that works your glutes, hamstrings and quads, and at the same time stretches the deep piriformis muscle in your butt.

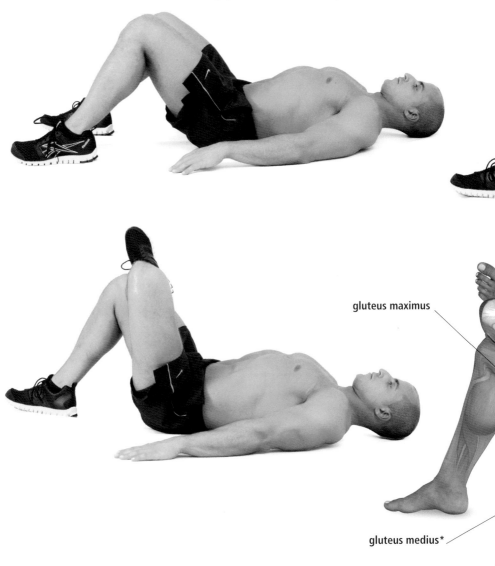

gluteus maximus

gluteus medius*

gluteus minimus*

HOW TO DO IT

1 Lie on your back, arms extended at your sides. Your knees should be bent, with feet on the floor.

2 Keeping the rest of your body still, raise your left leg to rest the ankle on your right knee.

3 Press your palms into the floor and engage your abdominal muscles as you lift. Your body from shoulders to knees should form a diagonal line.

4 Slowly and with control, return to starting position. Switch legs and repeat. Aim for 5 repetitions per side.

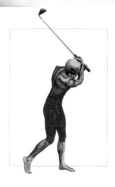

PRIMARY TARGETS
- gluteus maximus
- gluteus medius*
- gluteus minimus*
- biceps femoris
- semitendinosus
- semimembranosus
- rectus femoris
- vastus lateralis
- vastus intermedius*
- vastus medialis

BENEFITS
- Stretches piriformis
- Strengthens quadriceps, hamstrings and gluteal muscles

CAUTIONS
- Avoid tensing your neck.
- Lifting your shoulders toward your ears.

PERFECT YOUR FORM
- Squeeze your buttocks as you lift and lower.
- Draw your navel toward your spine.
- Press your shoulders down toward your back.

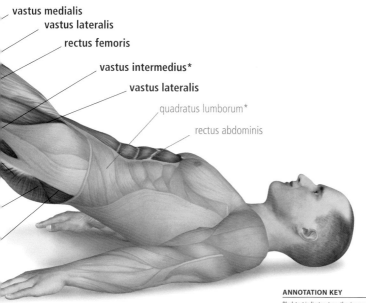

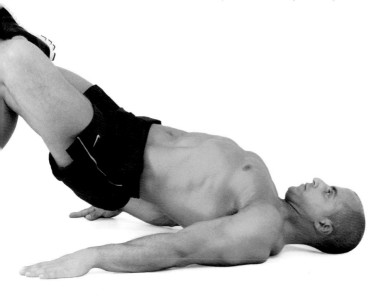

vastus medialis

vastus lateralis

rectus femoris

vastus intermedius*

vastus lateralis

quadratus lumborum*

rectus abdominis

ANNOTATION KEY

Black text indicates strengthening muscles
Gray text indicates stretching muscles
Italic text indicates tendons and ligaments
- - - - *indicates deep muscles

LATERAL EXTENSION LATERAL LUNGE

BEGINNER

THIS IS A GREAT exercise for people with short or stiff adductors, but it is an easy exercise to get wrong—many people make the mistake of stepping to the left or right and allowing their knee to translate too far forward over their toes. The knee is obviously going to come forward slightly, but the heel should stay down, planted on to the floor at all times.

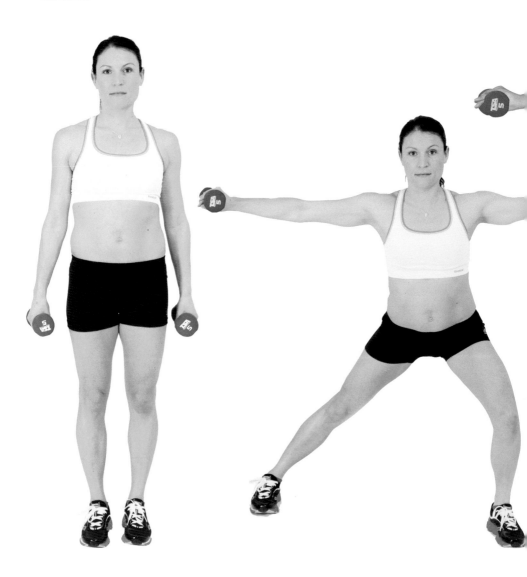

HOW TO DO IT

1 Stand with your feet hip-width apart and your arms at your sides, a dumbbell in each hand.

2 Take a big step to the left, and then bend your left knee to assume a side lunge position. At the same time, raise both arms so that they are parallel to the floor, forming a straight line.

3 Smoothly and with control, return to the starting position.

4 Repeat on the other side, working up to 10 repetitions on alternating sides.

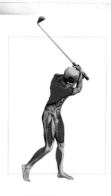

PRIMARY TARGETS
- trapezius
- rhomboideus*
- gluteus minimus*
- gluteus medius*
- gluteus maximus
- deltoideus medialis

BENEFITS
- Strengthens and tones shoulders and legs

CAUTIONS
- Avoid positioning one arm in front of the other in the raised position.

PERFECT YOUR FORM
- Keep your torso facing forward as you lunge to the side.
- Pull your abdominal muscles inward.

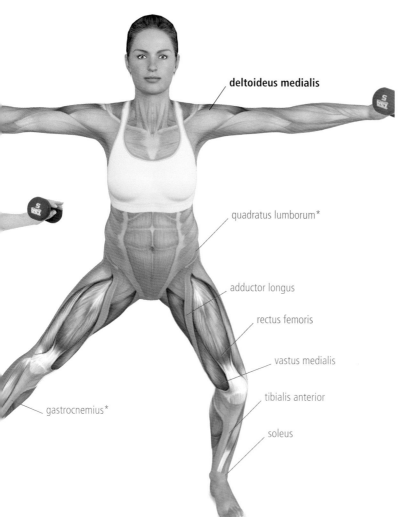

deltoideus medialis

quadratus lumborum*

adductor longus

rectus femoris

vastus medialis

tibialis anterior

gastrocnemius*

soleus

ANNOTATION KEY

Black text indicates strengthening muscles
Gray text indicates stretching muscles
Italic text indicates tendons and ligaments
- - - - *indicates deep muscles

KNEE-TO-CHEST HUG

BEGINNER

YOU DON'T EVEN need to get out of bed to do this stretch. Any time you find yourself relaxing on your back, incorporate this stretch. With the pull of gravity, the back, hip and groin muscles get a great stretch with not much effort.

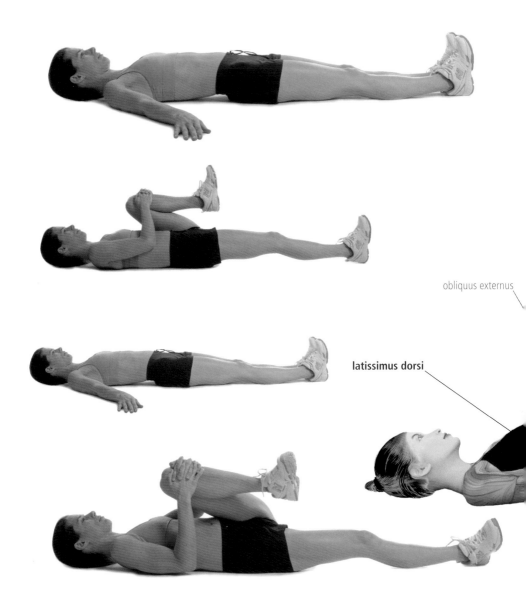

obliquus externus

latissimus dorsi

HOW TO DO IT

1 Lie supine on a mat with your legs together and arms outstretched.

2 Bend your right knee, and bring your foot to your body's midline while clasping your hands together to hold your knee. Hold the stretch for 15 seconds.

3 Return to the starting position.

4 Again, clasping your hands together to hold your knee, bend your right knee, but this time rotate the right leg to the left, bringing the side of your leg against your chest.

5 Hold the stretch for 15 seconds, and then return to the starting position. Repeat the entire sequence with the left leg bent.

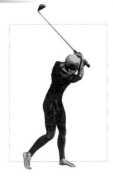

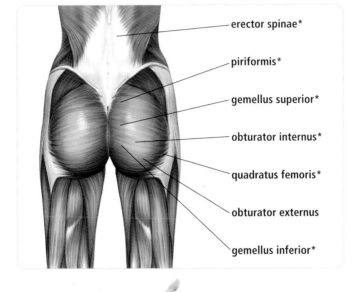

erector spinae*

piriformis*

gemellus superior*

obturator internus*

quadratus femoris*

obturator externus

gemellus inferior*

PRIMARY TARGETS
- erector spinae
- latissimus dorsi
- gluteus maximus
- gluteus minimus
- piriformis
- gemellus superior
- gemellus inferior
- obturator externus
- obturator internus
- quadratus femoris

BENEFITS
- Lower back
- Hips

CAUTIONS
- Avoid lifting your buttocks off the floor.

PERFECT YOUR FORM
- Keep your spine in neutral.

ANNOTATION KEY

Black text indicates strengthening muscles
Gray text indicates stretching muscles
Italic text indicates tendons and ligaments
- - - - *indicates deep muscles

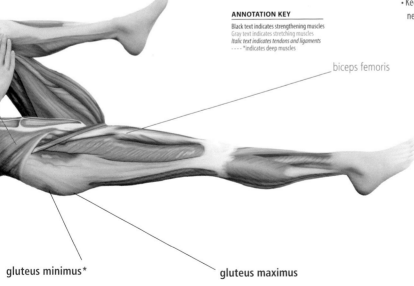

biceps femoris

gluteus minimus*

gluteus maximus

HIP ABDUCTION AND ADDUCTION

INTERMEDIATE

THE HIP ABDUCTION exercise performed with a resistance band around the ankle increases strength around your glute muscles. You will feel the exercise "burn" deep in your glutes. The resistance band places more demand on the muscles and triggers more strength development.

For hip adduction, stand in front of a low pulley inner, using a thigh machine; using ankle weights; or, as illustrated here, with an exercise band.

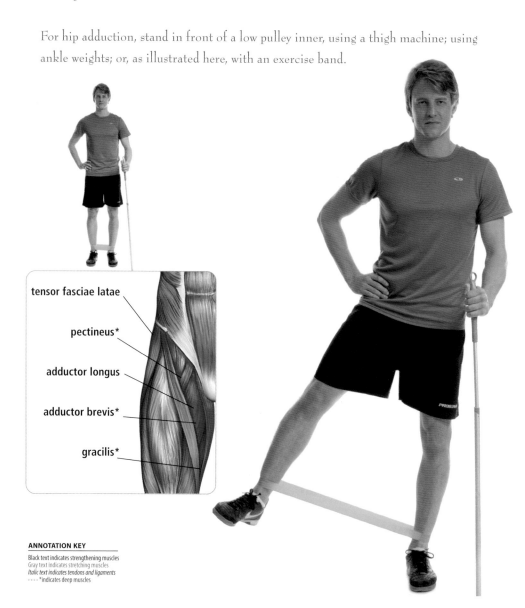

tensor fasciae latae

pectineus*

adductor longus

adductor brevis*

gracilis*

ANNOTATION KEY
Black text indicates strengthening muscles
Gray text indicates stretching muscles
Italic text indicates tendons and ligaments
- - - - *indicates deep muscles

HOW TO DO IT

1 Stand with your feet shoulder-width apart, with a resistance loop or a resistance band tied around your ankles. Tuck your pelvis slightly forward, lift your chest and press your shoulders downward and back. With your left hand, hold onto a support such as a mop handle or chair back.

2 Keeping your back and knee straight and foot facing forward, move your right foot directly to the right, moving away from your body. Hold for 2 seconds and repeat 10 times. Return to starting position.

1 Keeping your back and knee straight and foot facing forward, move your left foot directly to the right, moving it towards and across your body. Hold for 2 seconds and repeat 10 times.

2 Return to starting position, and repeat entire sequence on the opposite side.

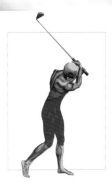

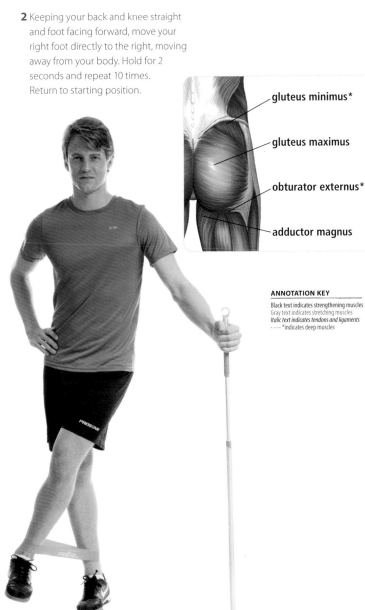

gluteus minimus*

gluteus maximus

obturator externus*

adductor magnus

ANNOTATION KEY

Black text indicates strengthening muscles
Gray text indicates stretching muscles
Italic text indicates tendons and ligaments
- - - - *indicates deep muscles

PRIMARY TARGETS

• adductor longus
• adductor magnus
• adductor brevis
• gracilis
• pectineus
• obturator externus
• gluteus minimus
• tensor fasciae latae
• gluteus maximus

BENEFITS

• Hip abductors
• Hip adductors

CAUTIONS

• Avoid touching your moving foot to the floor as you move your foot sideways and inward.

PERFECT YOUR FORM

• Tighten the muscles at the side of your thigh and hip as you move your leg.

SWIMMING

INTERMEDIATE

WHEN FIRST PRACTICING this exercise, you may feel like you aren't getting too far off the floor. If you try to lift up and feel a crunch in the lower back it means you have gone too far. Keep a balance between lifting up and extending out through the top of your head and toes.

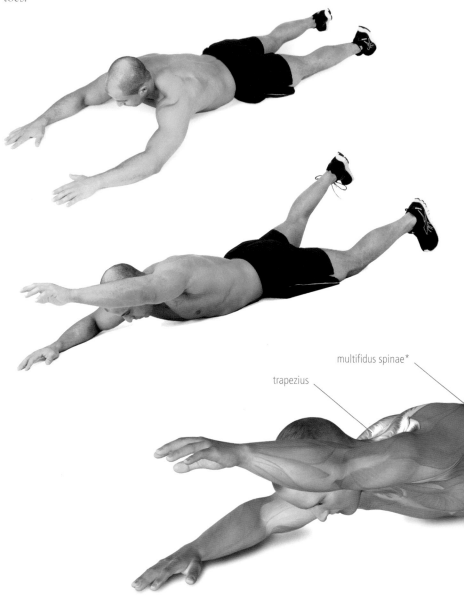

multifidus spinae*

trapezius

HOW TO DO IT

1 Lie on your stomach with your legs hip-width apart. Stretch your arms beside your ears on the floor. Engage your pelvic floor, and draw your navel into your spine.

2 Lift your right arm and left leg simultaneously. Raise your head slightly off the floor.

3 Lower your arm and leg to the starting position, maintaining a stretch in your limbs.

4 Repeat on the other side. Aim for 8 repetitions.

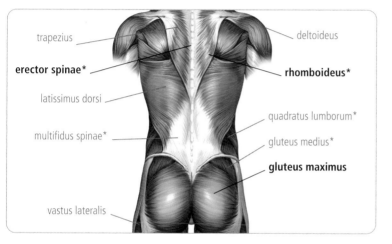

trapezius

deltoideus

erector spinae*

rhomboideus*

latissimus dorsi

quadratus lumborum*

multifidus spinae*

gluteus medius*

gluteus maximus

vastus lateralis

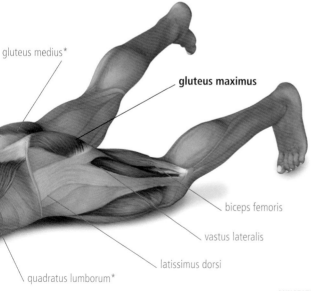

gluteus medius*

gluteus maximus

biceps femoris

vastus lateralis

latissimus dorsi

quadratus lumborum*

PRIMARY TARGETS
- rhomboideus*
- gluteus maximus
- erector spinae*

BENEFITS
- Stabilises core
- Tones abdominal muscles
- Strengthens hip and spinal extensors

CAUTIONS
- Avoid tensing your neck.
- Lifting your shoulders toward your ears.

PERFECT YOUR FORM
- Extend your upper back as you lift your arm and leg.
- Extend your limbs as long as possible in opposite directions.
- Keep your glutes tightly squeezed.

ANNOTATION KEY

Black text indicates strengthening muscles
Gray text indicates stretching muscles
Italic text indicates tendons and ligaments
- - - - *indicates deep muscles

LATERAL BAND SIDE STEPS

BEGINNER

ALTHOUGH THE LATERAL BAND SIDE STEPS exercise looks and feels strange at first, this exercise is a perfect way to improve hip stability, strengthen the hip—particularly the glutes—and increase the stability of the knee joint. This, in turn, improves overall body mechanics and movement efficiency.

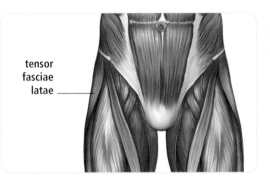

tensor fasciae latae

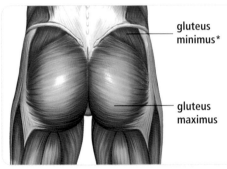

gluteus minimus*

gluteus maximus

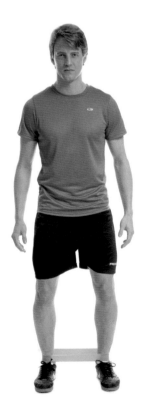

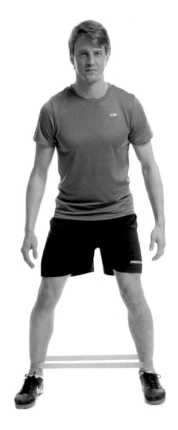

HOW TO DO IT

1 Stand with your feet shoulder-width apart, with a resistance loop or a resistance band tied around your ankles. Tuck your pelvis slightly forward, lift your chest and press your shoulders downward and back.

2 Keeping your head up, shoulders back, place your hands on your hips, and step sideways as far as you can while keeping your knees slightly bent and your posture tall.

3 Bring the opposite foot inward to meet the other foot, moving slowly and under control.

4 Continue to step to the side for one to three sets of 8 to 12 repetitions, then repeat in the other direction.

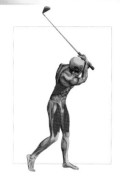

ANNOTATION KEY

Black text indicates strengthening muscles
Gray text indicates stretching muscles
Italic text indicates tendons and ligaments
- - - - *indicates deep muscles

PRIMARY TARGETS
• gluteus minimus*
• tensor fasciae latae
• gluteus maximus

BENEFITS
• Hip adductors

CAUTIONS
• Avoid leaning your torso to one side.

PERFECT YOUR FORM
• Tighten the muscles at the side of your thigh and hip as you move your leg.

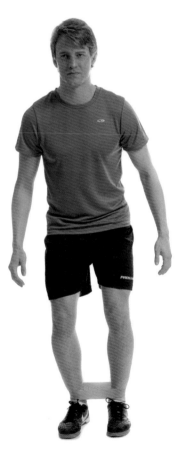

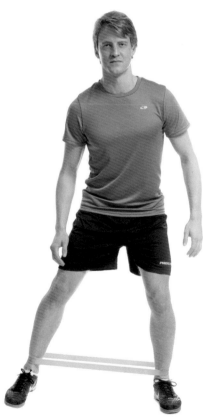

CROSSOVER STEPS

BEGINNER

As with the hip adduction exercise (page 199), this exercise can also be performed with ankle weights. It primarily works the collective muscles of your inner thighs and should be avoided by anyone with severe hip pain.

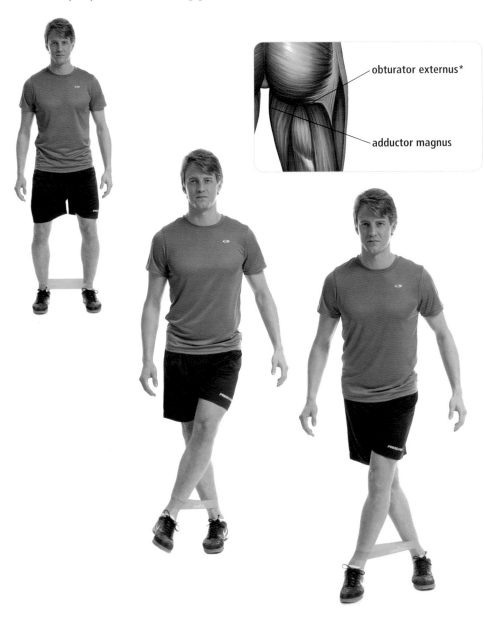

obturator externus*

adductor magnus

HOW TO DO IT

1 Stand with your feet shoulder-width apart, with a resistance loop or a resistance band tied around your ankles. Tuck your pelvis slightly forward, lift your chest and press your shoulders downwards and back.

2 Step out with your left foot until you feel moderate tension in the band, and then cross your left foot over your right.

3 Next, step your right foot in front of your left, and then step your left foot out, for a total of three steps with both feet to the left.

4 Return to the starting position, and then begin crossing right over left in the opposite direction.

5 Repeat all moves for a total of three sets in each direction.

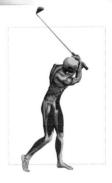

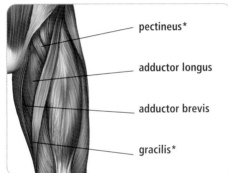

pectineus*

adductor longus

adductor brevis

gracilis*

ANNOTATION KEY
Black text indicates strengthening muscles
Gray text indicates stretching muscles
Italic text indicates tendons and ligaments
- - - - *indicates deep muscles

PRIMARY TARGETS
- adductor longus
- adductor magnus
- adductor brevis*
- gracilis
- pectineus
- obturator externus

BENEFITS
- Hip adductors

CAUTIONS
- Avoid rotating your torso.

PERFECT YOUR FORM
- Flex the toes of the moving foot toward your shin.
- Keep your hips square and pointed forward.
- Move at a pace that allows you to keep your balance.

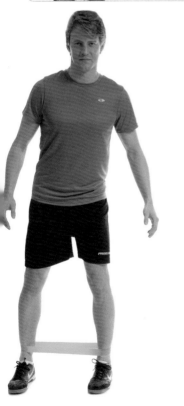

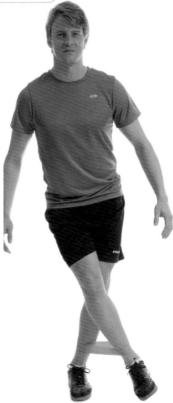

OBSTACLE CHALLENGE

INTERMEDIATE

The Obstacle Challenge benefit the glutes, quadriceps, hamstrings and calves. They help you practice lateral movement at speed. An easier variation is to complete a set of jumps to one side, and then switch. On the other hand, you can make the routine more difficult by adding more—or larger—cones.

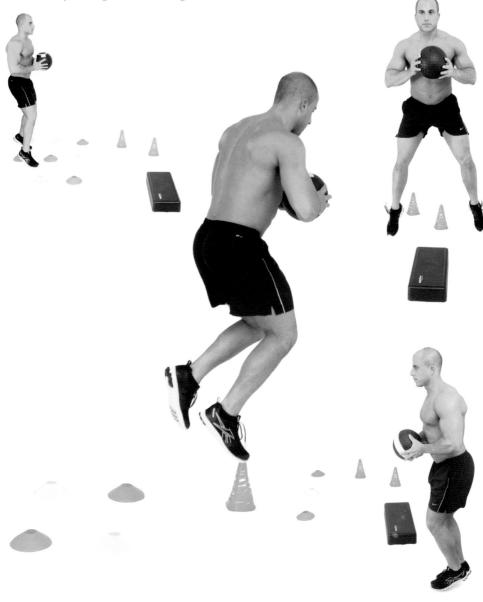

HOW TO DO IT

1 Set up a series of cones, shorter objects and a step on the floor as shown. Hold a medicine ball in front of your chest.

2 Jump between the objects as you make your way diagonally from one corner to the other.

3 Jump over one cone and then the other.

4 Still holding the ball, challenge yourself to jump over the step.

5 Jog back from the step to the beginning of the course. Begin again, completing the course up to 10 times.

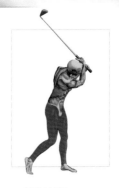

PRIMARY TARGETS
- rectus femoris
- vastus lateralis
- vastus intermedius*
- vastus medialis

BENEFITS
- Improves agility and flexibility
- Stabilises core

CAUTIONS
- Avoid twisting your neck.

PERFECT YOUR FORM
- Keep the medicine ball in place and centered in front of your chest.

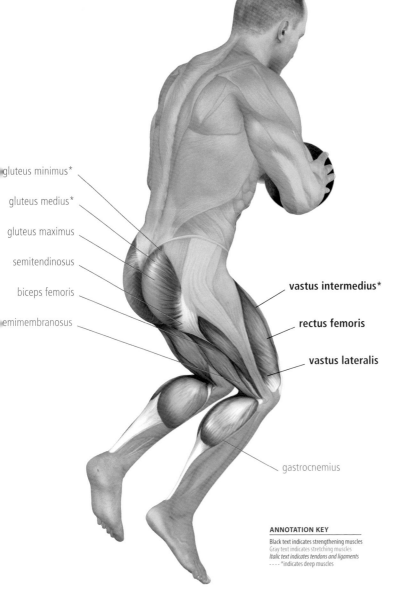

gluteus minimus*

gluteus medius*

gluteus maximus

semitendinosus

biceps femoris

semimembranosus

vastus intermedius*

rectus femoris

vastus lateralis

gastrocnemius

ANNOTATION KEY

Black text indicates strengthening muscles
Gray text indicates stretching muscles
Italic text indicates tendons and ligaments
- - - - *indicates deep muscles

STANDING KNEE CRUNCH

INTERMEDIATE

To SCULPT YOUR ABS, you'll need to exercise your obliques, the muscles that run down the sides of your stomach from your ribs to your hipbones. Standing Knee Crunches are a challenging exercise, requiring balance as well as stamina. They work your obliques, abs and glutes.

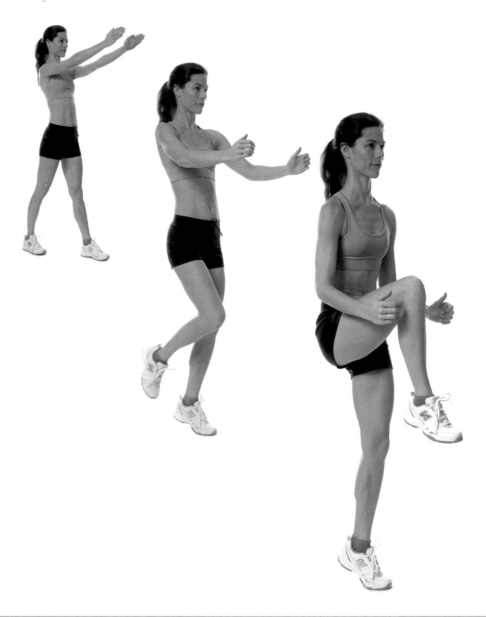

HOW TO DO IT

1 Stand tall with your left leg in front of the right, and extend your hands up toward the ceiling, your arms straight.

2 Shift your weight onto your left foot, and raise your right knee to the height of your hips. Simultaneously go up on the toes of your left leg, while pulling your elbows down by your sides, your hands making fists. This creates the crunch.

3 Pause at the top of the movement, and then return to the starting position. Repeat the sequence with your right leg as the standing leg. Repeat 10 times on each leg.

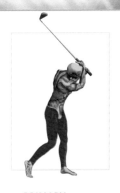

ANNOTATION KEY

Black text indicates strengthening muscles
Gray text indicates stretching muscles
Italic text indicates tendons and ligaments
- - - - *indicates deep muscles

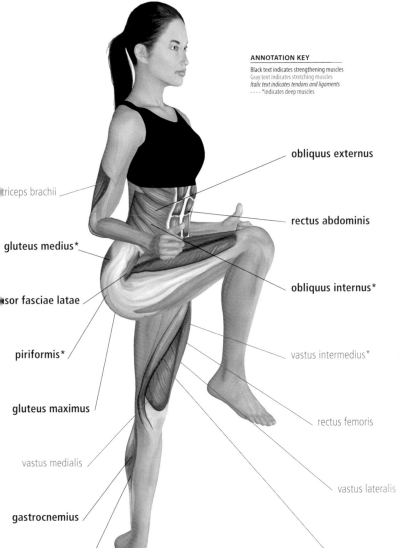

obliquus externus

rectus abdominis

obliquus internus*

vastus intermedius*

rectus femoris

vastus lateralis

sartorius

triceps brachii

gluteus medius*

sor fasciae latae

piriformis*

gluteus maximus

vastus medialis

gastrocnemius

soleus

PRIMARY TARGETS

- rectus abdominis
- obliquus internus
- obliquus externus
- transversus abdominis
- gluteus maximus
- gluteus medius
- tensor fasciae latae
- piriformis
- iliopsoas
- gastrocnemius
- soleus

BENEFITS

- Pelvic and core stabilisers
- Abdominals
- Gluteal area
- Calves

CAUTIONS

- Avoid tilting forward as you switch legs.

PERFECT YOUR FORM

- Keep your standing leg straight as you raise up on your toes.
- Relax your shoulders as you pull your arms down for the crunch.
- Flex the toes of your raised leg.

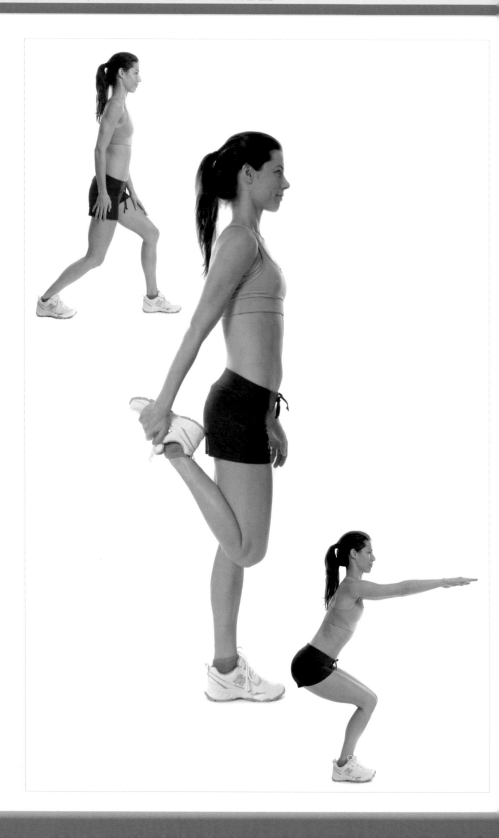

GOLF WORKOUTS

Once you have gone through the stretching and strengthening exercises in this book and practised executing them properly, your next step is to put these moves together. The following sequences are just samples of the many ways that you can combine these exercises to create golf training warm-ups and cool-downs, as well as targeted or all-over strengthening workouts. They provide flexible frameworks that you can adapt to accommodate your specific fitness level or area of concern—if you want to avoid a certain exercise in any one of them, simply substitute another that has a similar benefit. Try the workouts featured here, adding them to your training schedule workout days, and then flip through the exercises and create your own stretching routines and strengthening and stability workouts to suit your individual goals.

STRETCHES

A stretching routine offers many benefits, for the mind as well as the body. By following a stretching routine you can create elongated muscles, improve muscular coordination, increase flexibility, build up cardio endurance, boost energy and reduce stress. Stretching routines can also help with joint pain and lower back pain—a common complaint among golfers.

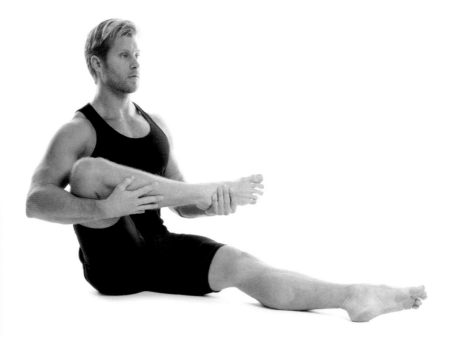

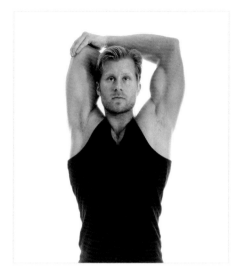

Triceps Stretch
page 36

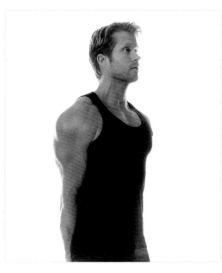

Biceps Stretch
page 38

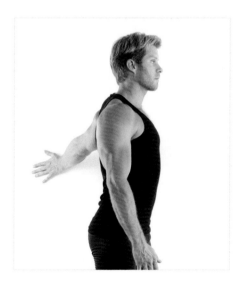

Wall-Assisted Chest Stretch
page 40

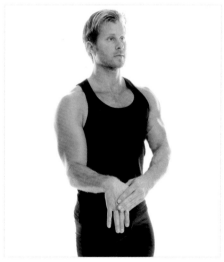

Wrist Flexion
page 44

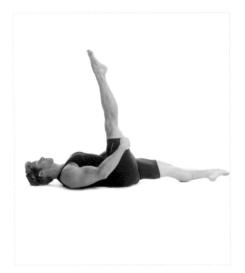

Unilateral Leg Stretch
page 102

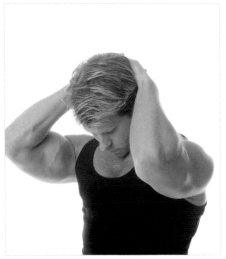

Neck Stretches
page 64

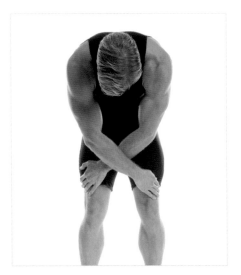

Standing Back Roll
page 66

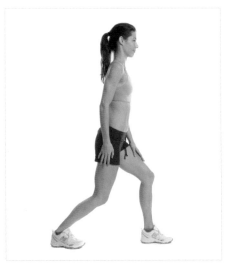

Gastrocnemius Stretch
page 106

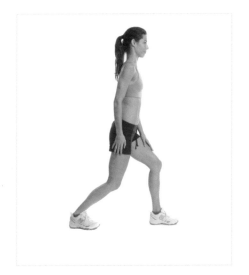

Soleus Stretch

page 108

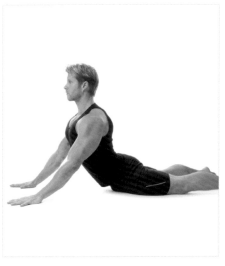

Cobra

page 144

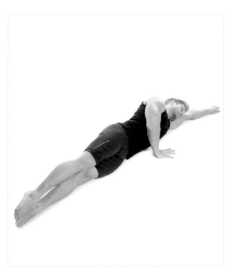

Side-Lying Knee Bend

page 94

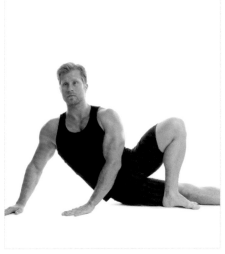

Side-Lying Rib Stretch

page 146

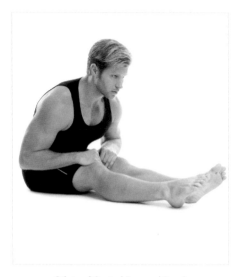

Bilateral Seated Forward Bend

page 104

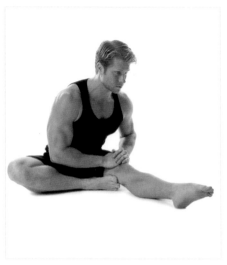

Unilateral Seated Forward Bend

page 100

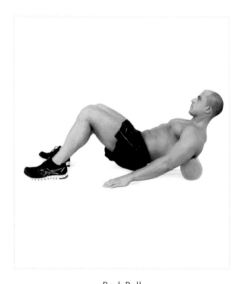

Back Roll

page 82

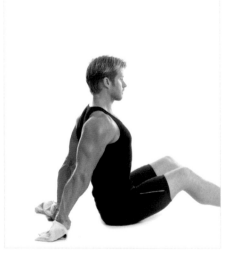

Front Deltoid Towel Stretch

page 42

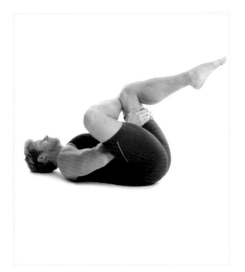

Lying Down Figure 4

page 182

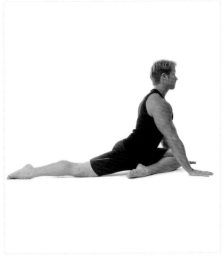

Pigeon Stretch

page 180

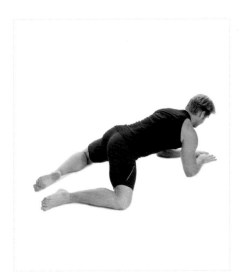

Frog Straddle

page 98

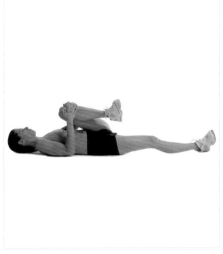

Knee-to-Chest Hug

page 196

PAR WORKOUTS

This workout is aimed at beginners. Perform three workouts per week, resting at least a day between each. You'll need to set aside half an hour for each workout. Perform the exercises as a group. Do one set of nine repetitions of each exercise, and rest for one minute between each exercise. Stay on this program for six weeks, adding 2 extra sets per week.

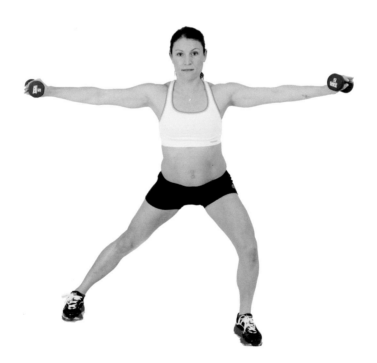

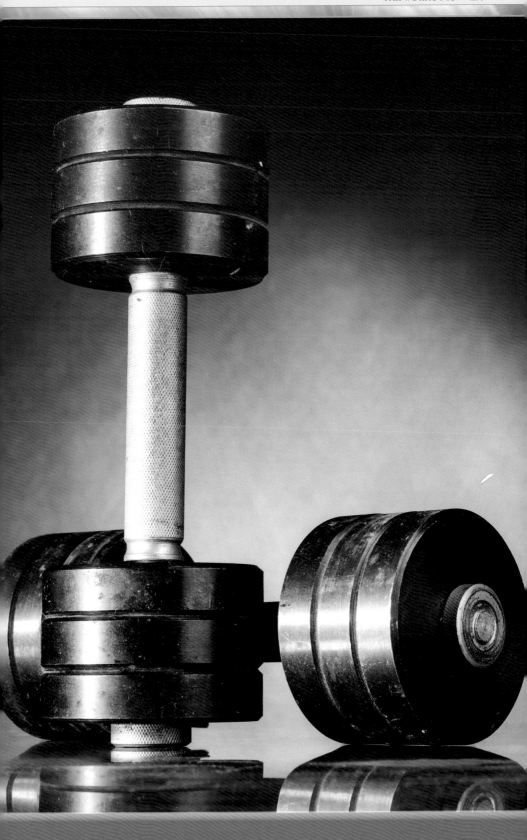

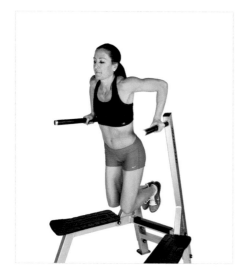

Dips

page 46

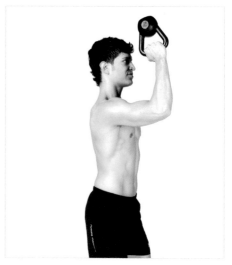

Bottoms-Up Kettlebell Clean

page 48

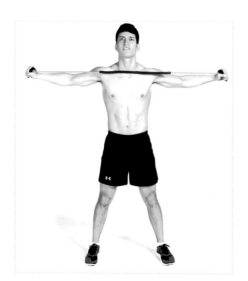

Band Pull-Apart

page 50

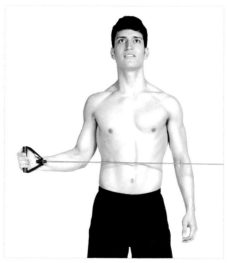

External Rotation with Band

page 52

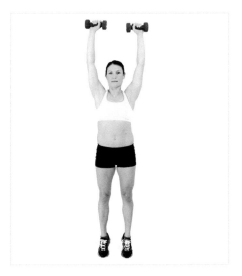

Heel Raise with Overhead Press
page 54

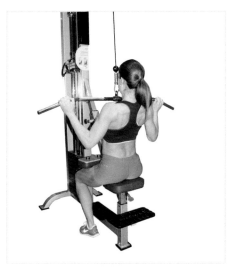

Lat Pulldowns
page 70

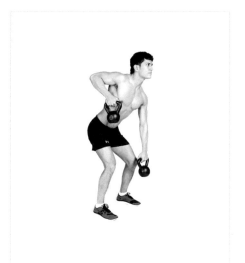

Alternating Kettlebell Row
page 72

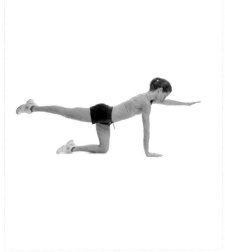

Quadruped Leg Lift
page 84

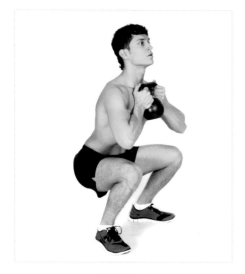

Goblet Squat

page 110

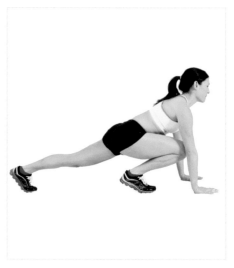

Mountain Climber

page 120

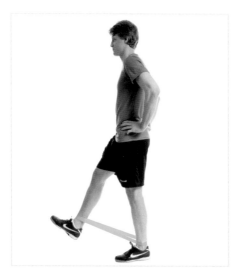

Hip Extension and Flexion

page 126

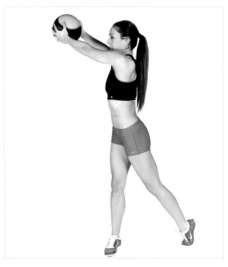

Medicine Ball Woodchop

page 152

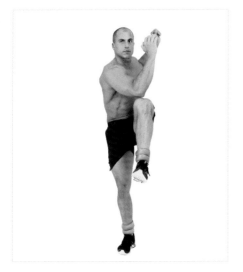

Twisting Knee Raise

page 160

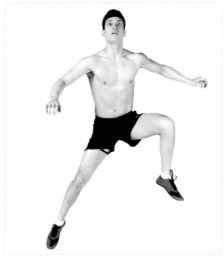

Lateral Bounding

page 188

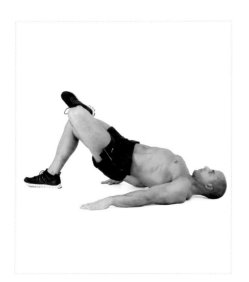

Piriformis Bridge

page 192

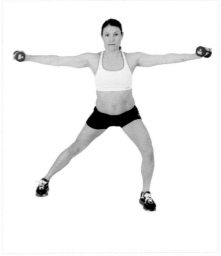

Lateral Extension Lateral Lunge

page 194

BIRDIE WORKOUTS

O nce you have finished the "Par" program, you can move on to this intermediate routine. Perform three workouts per week, resting at least a day between each. You'll need to set aside 45 minutes for each workout. Perform the exercises as a group. Do one set of eighteen repetitions of each exercise, and rest for one minute between each exercise. Stay on this program for six weeks.

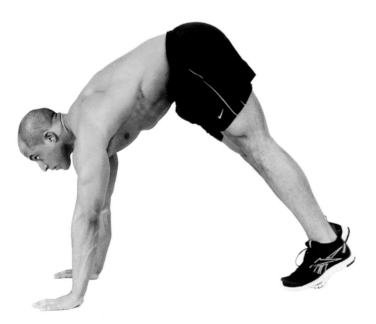

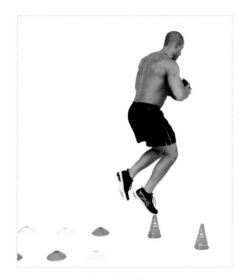

Obstacle Challenge
page 206

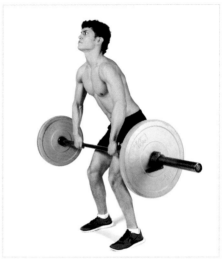

Barbell Power Clean
page 78

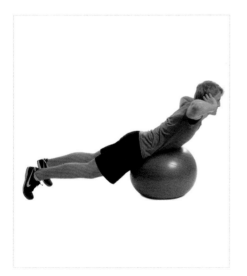

Swiss Ball Extension
page 86

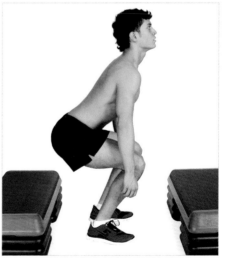

Depth Jumps
page 112

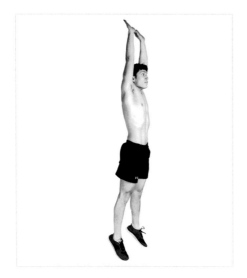

Burpees

page 114

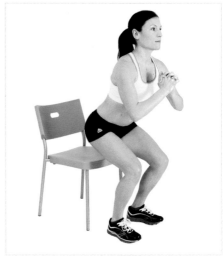

Chair Squat

page 118

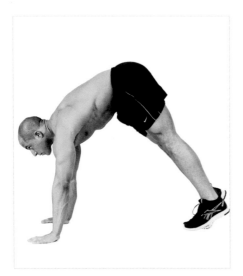

Push-Up Walkout

page 156

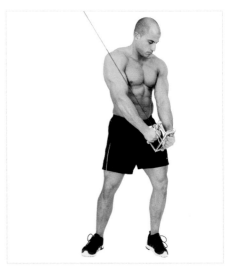

Twisting Lift

page 162

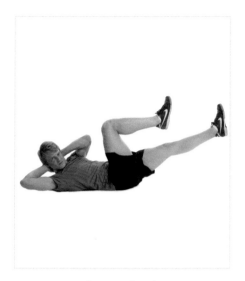

Crossover Crunch

page 164

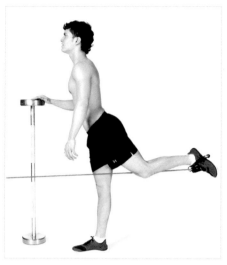

Hip Extension with Band

page 186

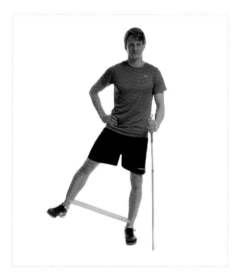

Hip Abduction and Adduction

page 198

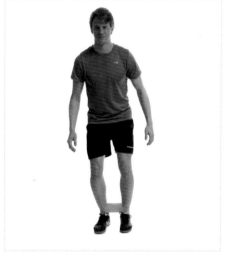

Lateral Band Side Steps

page 202

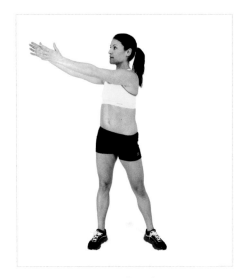

Diagonal Reach

page 166

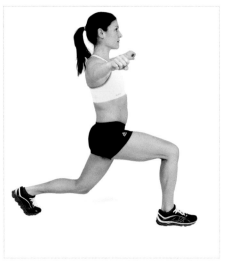

Lateral Extension Reverse Lunge

page 128

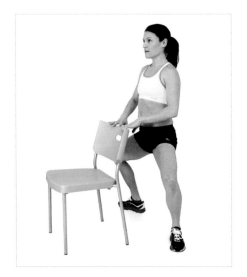

Chair Plié

page 130

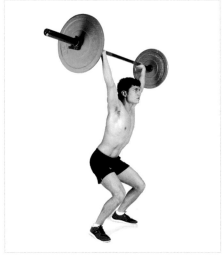

Barbell Squat

page 132

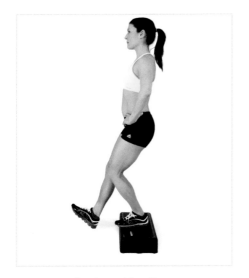

One-Legged Step Down
page 138

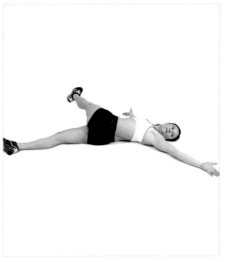

Full Body Roll
page 80

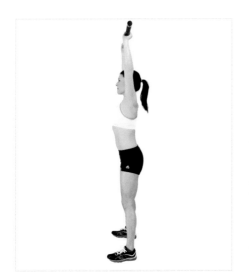

Clean and Lift
page 88

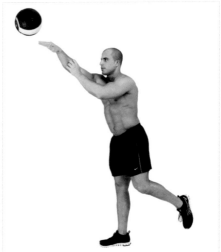

Knee-Flexion Ball Throw
page 174

EAGLE WORKOUTS

Once you have finished the "Birdie" program you can move on to this advanced routine. Perform three workouts per week, resting at least a day between each. You'll need to set aside an hour for each workout. Perform the exercises as a group. Do two set of eighteen repetitions of each exercise, rest for 45 seconds between each exercise and for three minutes for each set.

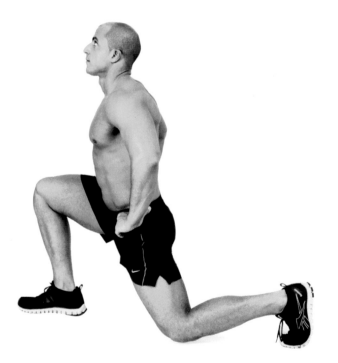

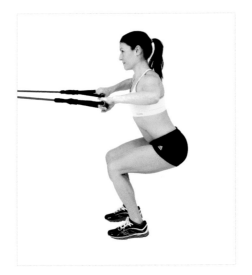

Squat and Row

page 56

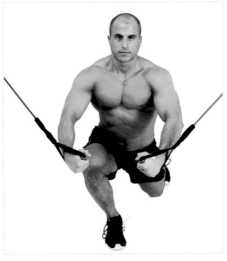

Reverse Lunge with Chest Press

page 58

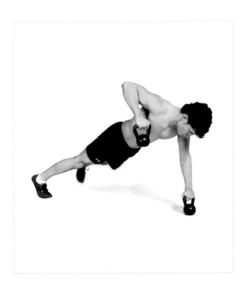

Alternating Renegade Row

page 74

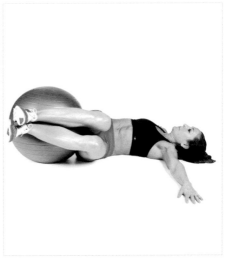

Swiss Ball Hip Crossover

page 76

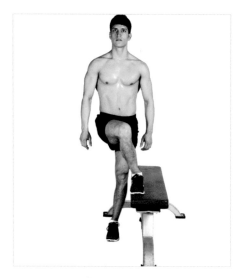

Crossover Stepup
page 116

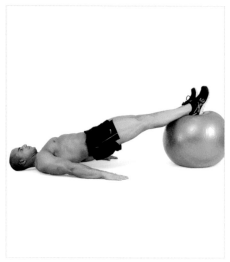

Swiss Ball Bridging Raise
page 122

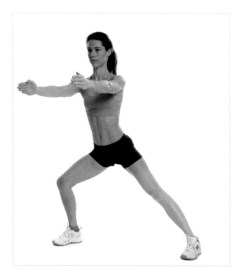

Lateral Low Lunge
page 124

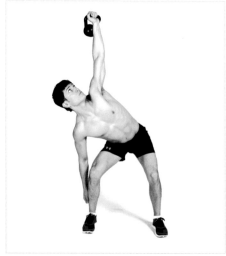

Advanced Kettlebell Windmill
page 148

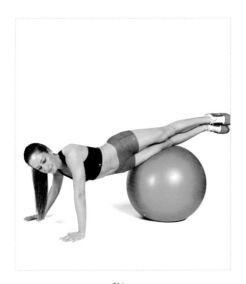

Skier

page 150

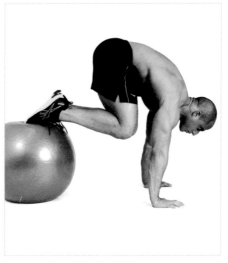

Swiss Ball Jack Knife

page 154

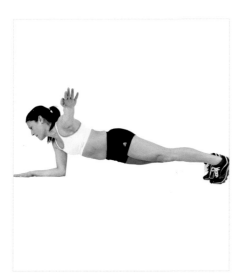

Arm-Reach Plank

page 158

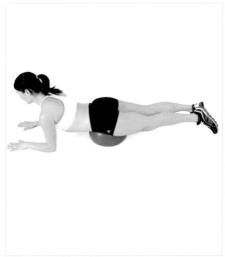

Heel Beats

page 190

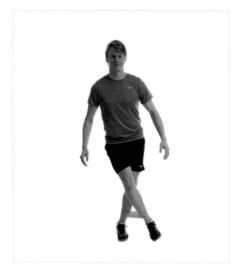

Crossover Steps
page 204

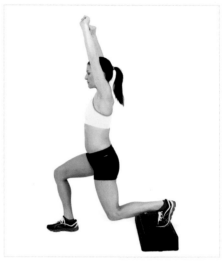

Split Squat with Overhead Press
page 134

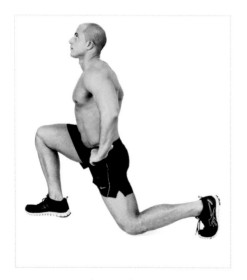

Jumping Lunge
page 136

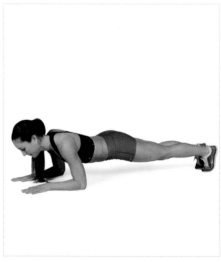

Plank
page 170

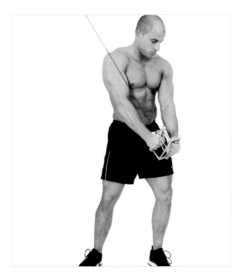

Woodchop

page 172

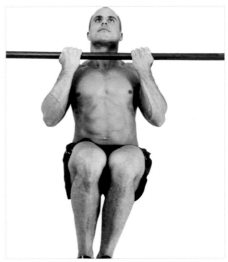

Chin-Up with Hanging Leg Raise

page 60

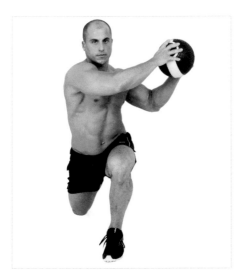

Reach-and-Twist Walking Lunge

page 140

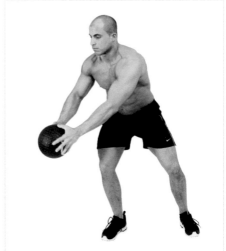

Figure 8

page 176

GLOSSARY

GENERAL TERMS

abduction: Movement away from the body.

adduction: Movement toward the body.

aerobic step: A portable step or platform with adjustable risers designed for cardiovascular exercising that also allows you to effectively work your calf muscles.

agonist muscle: See *antagonist muscle*.

anterior: Located in the front.

antagonist muscle: A muscle working in opposition to another, called the *agonist*. Most muscles work in antagonistic pairs, with one muscle contracting as the other expands; for example, when the biceps brachii contracts, the triceps brachii relaxes.

cardiovascular exercise: Any exercise that increases the heart rate, making oxygen and nutrient-rich blood available to muscles.

core: Refers to the deep muscle layers that lie close to the spine and provide structural support for the entire body. The core is divisible into two groups: the major core and the minor core. The major muscles reside on the trunk and include the belly area and the mid and lower back. This area encompasses the pelvic floor muscles (levator ani, pubococcygeus, iliococcygeus, puborectalis, and coccygeus), the abdominals (rectus abdominis, transversus abdominis, obliquus externus, and obliquus internus), the spinal extensors (multifidus spinae, erector spinae, splenius, longissimus thoracis, and semispinalis) and the diaphragm. The minor core muscles include the latissimus dorsi, gluteus maximus and trapezius. Minor core muscles assist the major muscles when the body engages in activities or movements that require added stability.

crunch: A common abdominal exercise that calls for curling the shoulders toward the pelvis while lying supine with hands behind the head and knees bent.

curl: An exercise movement, usually targeting the biceps brachii, that calls for a weight to be moved through an arc, in a "curling" motion.

deadlift: An exercise movement that calls for lifting a weight, such as a dumbbell, off the floor from a stabilized bent-over position.

dumbbell: A basic piece of equipment that consists of a short bar on which plates are secured. A person can use a dumbbell in one or both hands during an exercise. Most gyms offer dumbbells with the weight plates welded on and poundage indicated on the plates, but many dumbbells intended for home use come with removable plates that allow you to adjust the weight.

extension: The act of straightening.

extensor muscle: A muscle serving to extend a body part away from the body.

flexion: The bending of a joint.

flexor muscle: A muscle that decreases the angle between two bones, as when bending the arm at the elbow or raising the thigh toward the stomach.

foam roller: A tube that comes in a variety of sizes, materials and densities that can be used for stretching, strengthening, balance training, stability training and self-massage.

gait cycle: The rhythmic alternating movements of the legs that result in the forward movement of the body, or the way we run or walk.

hamstrings: The three muscles of the posterior thigh (the semitendinosus, semimembranosus and biceps femoris) that work to flex the knee and extend the hip.

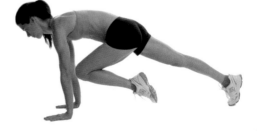

hand weight: Any of a range of free weights that are often used in weight training and toning. Small hand weights are usually cast iron formed in the shape of a dumbbell, sometimes coated with rubber or neoprene.

iliotibial band (ITB): A thick band of fibrous tissue that runs down the outside of the leg, beginning at the hip and extending to the outer side of the tibia just below the knee joint. The band functions in concert with several of the thigh muscles to provide stability to the outside of the knee joint.

lateral: Located on, or extending toward, the outside.

medial: Located on, or extending toward, the middle.

medicine ball: A small weighted ball used in weight training and toning.

neutral position (spine): A spinal position resembling an S shape, consisting of a inward curve in the lower back when viewed in profile.

posterior: Located behind.

press: An exercise movement that calls for moving a weight or other resistance away from the body.

primary muscle: One of the main muscles activated during a certain activity.

pronation: Turning inward. A pronated foot is one in which the heel bone angles inward and the arch tends to collapse. Opposite of *supination*.

quadriceps: A large muscle group (full name: quadriceps femoris) that includes the four prevailing muscles on the front of the thigh: the rectus femoris, vastus intermedius, vastus lateralis and vastus medialis. It is the great extensor muscle of the knee, forming a large fleshy mass that covers the front and sides of the femur muscle.

range of motion: The distance and direction a joint can move between the flexed position and the extended position.

resistance band: Any rubber tubing or flat band device that provides a resistive force used for strength training. Also called a "fitness band," "Thera-Band," "Dyna-Band," "stretching band" and "exercise band."

rotator muscle: One of a group of muscles that assist the rotation of a joint, such as the hip or the shoulder.

scapula: The protrusion of bone on the mid to upper back, also known as the "shoulder blade."

secondary muscle: A muscle activated during a certain activity that usually works to support the primary muscles.

squat: An exercise movement that calls for moving the hips back and bending the knees and hips to lower the torso and an accompanying weight, and then returning to the upright position. A squat primarily targets the muscles of the thighs, hips, buttocks and hamstrings.

supination: Turning outward. In running, supination is the insufficient inward roll of the foot after landing. This places extra stress on the foot and can result in iliotibial band syndrome, Achilles tendonitis or plantar fasciitis. Also know as "overpronation."

Swiss ball: A flexile, inflatable PVC ball measuring approximately 18 to 30 inches (45 to 75 cm) in diameter that is used for weight training, physical therapy, balance training and many other exercise regimens. It is also called a "balance ball," "fitness ball," "stability ball," "exercise ball," "gym ball," "physioball," "body ball," "therapy ball" and many other names.

warm-up: Any form of light exercise of short duration that prepares the body for more intense exercises.

weight: Refers to the plates or weight stacks, or the actual poundage listed on the bar or dumbbell.

LATIN TERMS

The following glossary explains the Latin scientific terminology used to describe the muscles of the human body. Certain words are derived from Greek, which is indicated in each instance.

CHEST

coracobrachialis: Greek *korakoeidés*, 'ravenlike,' and *brachium*, 'arm'

pectoralis (major and minor): *pectus*, 'breast'

ABDOMEN

obliquus externus: *obliquus*, 'slanting,' and *externus*, 'outward'

obliquus internus: *obliquus*, 'slanting,' and *internus*, 'within'

rectus abdominis: *rego*, 'straight, upright,' and *abdomen*, 'belly'

serratus anterior: *serra*, 'saw,' and *ante*, 'before'

transversus abdominis: *transversus*, 'athwart,' and *abdomen*, 'belly'

NECK

scalenus: Greek *skalénós*, 'unequal'

semispinalis: *semi*, 'half,' and *spinae*, 'spine'

splenius: Greek *spléníon*, 'plaster, patch'

sternocleidomastoideus: Greek *stérnon*, 'chest,' Greek *kleís*, 'key' and Greek *mastoeidés*, 'breastlike'

BACK

erector spinae: *erectus*, 'straight,' and *spina*, 'thorn'

latissimus dorsi: *latus*, 'wide,' and *dorsum*, 'back'

multifidus spinae: *multifid*, 'to cut into divisions,' and *spinae*, 'spine'

quadratus lumborum: *quadratus*, 'square, rectangular,' and *lumbus*, 'loin'

rhomboideus: Greek *rhembesthai*, 'to spin'

trapezius: Greek *trapezion*, 'small table'

SHOULDERS

deltoideus (anterior, medial, and posterior): Greek *deltoeidés*, 'delta-shaped'

infraspinatus: *infra*, 'under,' and *spina*, 'thorn'

levator scapulae: *levare*, 'to raise,' and *scapulae*, 'shoulder [blades]'

subscapularis: *sub*, 'below,' and *scapulae*, 'shoulder [blades]'

supraspinatus: *supra*, 'above,' and *spina*, 'thorn'

teres (major and minor): *teres*, 'rounded'

UPPER ARM

biceps brachii: *biceps*, 'two-headed,' and *brachium*, 'arm'

brachialis: *brachium*, 'arm'

triceps brachii: *triceps*, 'three-headed' and *brachium*, 'arm'

LOWER ARM

anconeus: Greek *anconad*, 'elbow'

brachioradialis: *brachium*, 'arm,' and *radius*, 'spoke'

extensor carpi radialis: *extendere*, 'to extend,' Greek *karpós*, 'wrist' and *radius*, 'spoke'

extensor digitorum: *extendere*, 'to extend,' and *digitus*, 'finger, toe'

flexor carpi pollicis longus: *flectere*, 'to bend,' Greek *karpós*, 'wrist,' *pollicis*, 'thumb' and *longus*, 'long'

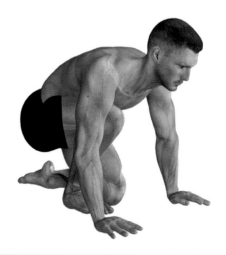

flexor carpi radialis: *flectere*, 'to bend,' Greek *karpós*, 'wrist' and *radius*, 'spoke'

flexor carpi ulnaris: *flectere*, 'to bend,' Greek *karpós*, 'wrist,' and *ulnaris*, 'forearm'

flexor digitorum: *flectere*, 'to bend,' and *digitus*, 'finger, toe'

palmaris longus: *palmaris*, 'palm,' and *longus*, 'long'

pronator teres: *pronate*, 'to rotate,' and *teres*, 'rounded'

HIPS

gemellus (inferior and superior): *geminus*, 'twin'

gluteus maximus: Greek *gloutós*, 'rump,' and *maximus*, 'largest'

gluteus medius: Greek *gloutós*, 'rump' and *medialis*, 'middle'

gluteus minimus: Greek *gloutós*, 'rump' and *minimus*, 'smallest'

iliopsoas: *ilium*, 'groin,' and Greek *psoa*, 'groin muscle'

obturator externus: *obturare*, 'to block' and *externus*, 'outward'

obturator internus: *obturare*, 'to block' and *internus*, 'within'

pectineus: *pectin*, 'comb'

piriformis: *pirum*, 'pear,' and *forma*, 'shape'

quadratus femoris: *quadratus*, 'square, rectangular,' and *femur*, 'thigh'

UPPER LEG

adductor longus: *adducere*, 'to contract,' and *longus*, 'long'

adductor magnus: *adducere*, 'to contract,' and *magnus*, 'major'

biceps femoris: *biceps*, 'two-headed,' and *femur*, 'thigh'

gracilis: *gracilis*, 'slim, slender'

rectus femoris: *rego*, 'straight, upright,' and *femur*, 'thigh'

sartorius: *sarcio*, 'to patch' or 'to repair'

semimembranosus: *semi*, 'half,' and *membrum*, 'limb'

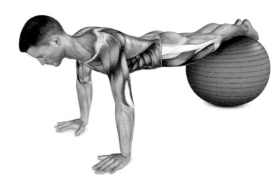

semitendinosus: *semi*, 'half,' and *tendo*, 'tendon'

tensor fasciae latae: *tenere*, 'to stretch,' *fasciae*, 'band,' and *latae*, 'laid down'

vastus intermedius: *vastus*, 'immense, huge,' and *intermedius*, 'between'

vastus lateralis: *vastus*, 'immense, huge,' and *lateralis*, 'side'

vastus medialis: *vastus*, 'immense, huge,' and *medialis*, 'middle'

LOWER LEG

adductor digiti minimi: *adducere*, 'to contract,' *digitus*, 'finger, toe,' and *minimum* 'smallest'

adductor hallucis: *adducere*, 'to contract,' and *hallex*, 'big toe'

extensor digitorum longus: *extendere*, 'to extend,' *digitus*, 'finger, toe' and *longus*, 'long'

extensor hallucis longus: *extendere*, 'to extend,' *hallex*, 'big toe,' and *longus*, 'long'

flexor digitorum longus: *flectere*, 'to bend,' *digitus*, 'finger, toe' and *longus*, 'long'

flexor hallucis longus: *flectere*, 'to bend,' and *hallex*, 'big toe' and *longus*, 'long'

gastrocnemius: Greek *gastroknémia*, 'calf [of the leg]'

peroneus: *peronei*, 'of the fibula'

plantaris: *planta*, 'the sole'

soleus: *solea*, 'sandal'

tibialis anterior: *tibia*, 'reed pipe,' and *ante*, 'before'

tibialis posterior: *tibia*, 'reed pipe,' and *posterus*, 'coming after'

CREDITS

Created by Adam Moore

Moseley Road Inc.
123 Main Street
Irvington, New York 10533

President: Sean Moore
Production & Art director: Adam Moore
Photographer: Jonathan Conklin Photography, Inc.

Illustrator: Hector Aiza/3D Labz Animation India (www.3dlabz.com)